"A First Book for Understanding Diabetes"
is a synopsis of the larger book,
"Understanding Diabetes."

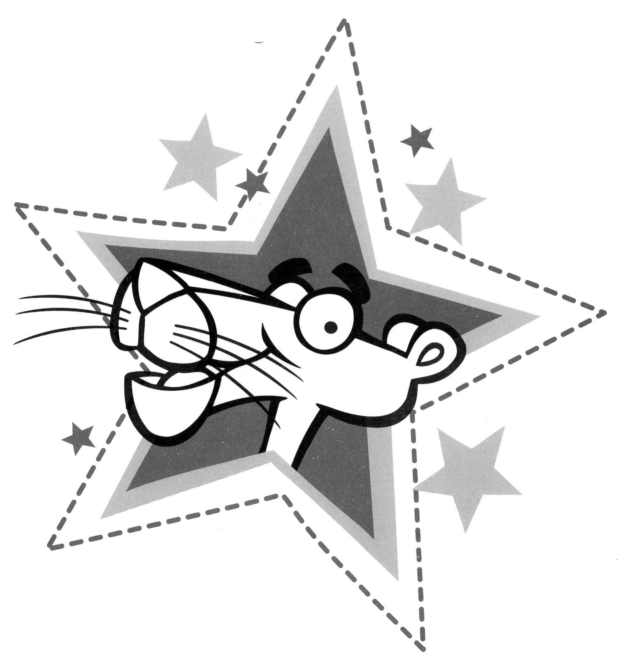

It provides a quick summary of each of the chapters.
It may be easier to begin learning from this book
until you are ready to read the larger book.

notes

14th Edition
A First Book for
UNDERSTANDING
Diabetes

"A First Book for Understanding Diabetes" is a synopsis of the larger book, "Understanding Diabetes"

Brigitte I. Frohnert, MD, PhD
and
H. Peter Chase, MD

Barbara Davis Center
for Diabetes

For information, contact:
Children's Diabetes Foundation
4380 South Syracuse Street, Suite 430
Denver, CO 80237

www.ChildrensDiabetesFoundation.org

Library of Congress Control Number 2018939213
ISBN 978-1-7320485-0-8

Published by
Children's Diabetes Foundation
4380 South Syracuse Street, Suite 430 Denver, CO 80237
303-863-1200

Book Design by Scott Johnson

Printed in the United States of America
by American Web

This book is dedicated
to the many parents and families
who do so much to care for their
children with diabetes.

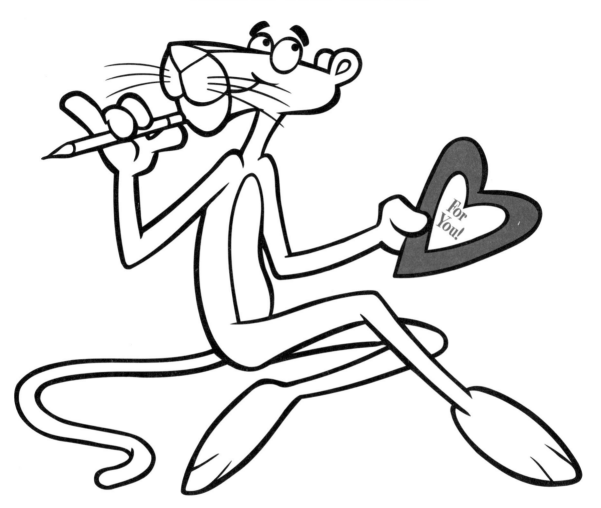

Special Thanks to...

The staff of the Children's Diabetes Foundation.

Mrs. Emily Fose for editing and proofreading.

Regina Reece for manuscript preparation and editing.

Scott Johnson for book design and graphics.

MGM Consumer Products for allowing the use of THE PINK PANTHER™.
www.pinkpanther.com

Additional copies of this publication may be purchased from
the Children's Diabetes Foundation.
See available publications at the end of this book.

Table of Contents

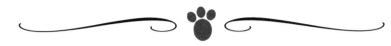

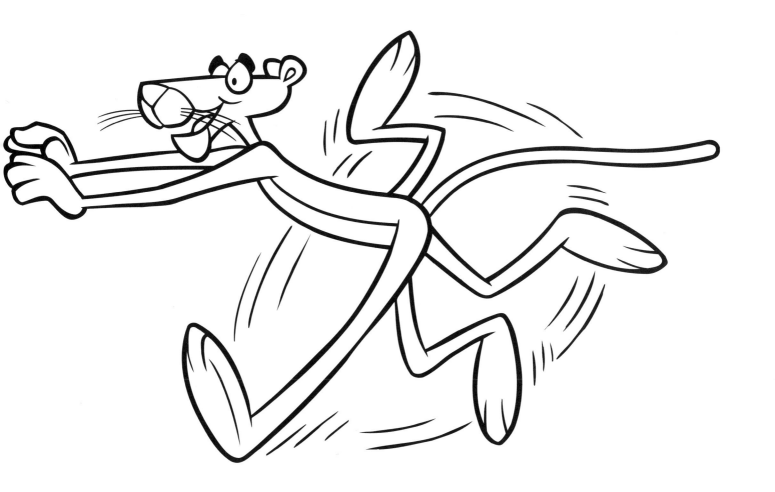

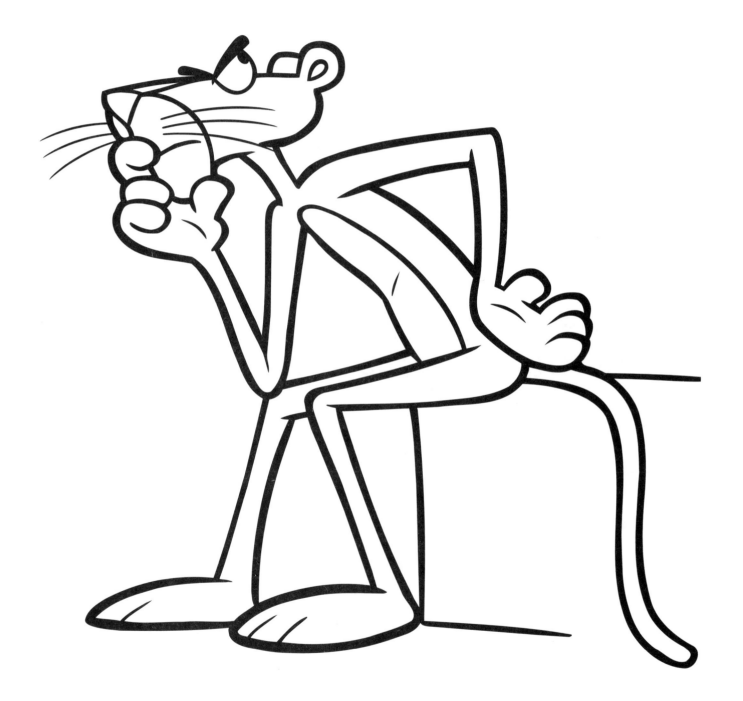

Chapter 1
The Importance of Education in Diabetes

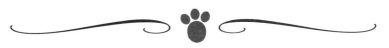

It is important to learn all about diabetes. At the time of diagnosis, the family will spend one to three days learning about diabetes. Early education will focus on initial survival skills. Approximately one week later, they will return for another day. This book will help in the beginning, until the family is ready to read the larger book, *"Understanding Diabetes."* In both books, the chapters have the same numbers and topics. All family members, including both parents, should be present for initial education. In this book we use "you" for you and your child.

Initial teaching (survival skills) often includes:

☐ What diabetes is and what causes it

☐ Urine and/or blood ketone checking

☐ Blood sugar/continuous glucose monitor (CGM) checking

☐ Recognizing a low blood sugar and how to treat it

☐ Insulin types and actions

☐ Drawing up insulin

☐ Giving shots

☐ Food survival skills

In addition to survival skills, other areas often covered are:

☐ A school plan

☐ When to call your diabetes care-provider

☐ Details of treatment (including "thinking" scales)

☐ Education about food (dietitian)

☐ Feelings (psych-social team)

☐ Plans for the next few days

One-Week Follow Up

Usually at one week, the family and child return for group education with other families. The content includes teaching done by the dietitian and nurse and a clinic visit with the physician, a nurse practitioner or physician assistant. Areas covered include:

☐ Details of food management with diabetes

☐ Review of HbA1c: what is it, why is it important

☐ Insulin actions and different insulin regimens

☐ Pattern management of blood/CGM sugars: how to identify trends and when to fax or email numbers (all families are given fax sheets to send in weekly until sugar levels and insulin doses stabilize)

☐ Low blood sugar care: causes, signs and treatment of mild to severe low blood sugars, including a review of the use of glucose tablets and gel and the administration of glucagon

☐ High blood/CGM sugar care: prevention of diabetic ketoacidosis; causes, signs and treatment

☐ Sick day management: how often to check blood sugars and ketones, fluid replacement — what type and how much, when and how to urgently call for assistance

The importance of
education in diabetes.

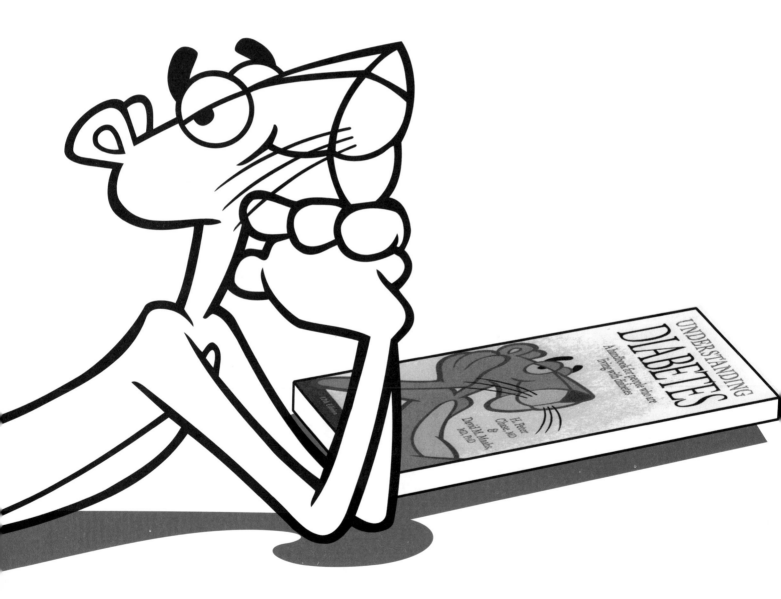

Special instructions for the first night are summarized below.

A. *The diabetes supplies you will need the first night include* (your nurse will mark which you need):

____ Blood glucose meter   ____ Meter glucose strips   ____ Alcohol swabs

____ Ketone check strips   ____ Glucose gel & tabs   ____ Log book

____ Insulin   ____ Syringes   ____ Phone card

The first night, either you will get your insulin injection at our Clinic, or you will give the shot at home or where you are staying.

B. *If the insulin is given while at the clinic:*

1. If Humalog® (Admelog)/NovoLog® or Apidra® insulin has been given, eat in 15-20 minutes (or have a snack if blood sugar below 100 mg/dL [<5.5 mmol/L]).

2. If Regular insulin has been given, try to eat your meal in 30 minutes – or have a snack containing carbohydrates if it will be more than 30 minutes.

3. Eat until the appetite is satisfied, avoiding high sugar foods (especially regular sugar pop [soda], other sweetened drinks, juice and sweet desserts).

C. *If the dinner insulin is to be given at home:*

1. Check the blood sugar right before the injection. Enter the result into the log book.

2. Check for urine ketones.

3. Call _____ at _____ or page at _____ for an insulin dose.
   Give this dose: _____.

4. Draw up and give the insulin injection 15-20 minutes before the meal (give at mealtime if below 100 mg/dL [<5.5 mmol/L]). If you are not very hungry, or are too tired to eat, call the diabetes care team with any dose questions.

D. *Before Bed:*

1. Check the blood sugar. Enter the result into the log book.

2. Check for urine or blood ketones.

3. Call your physician at the numbers listed above if the blood sugar is below ____ or above ____, or if urine ketones are "moderate" or "large" or if blood ketones are >0.6 mmol/L. If urine ketones are "trace" or "small," drink 8-12 oz of water before going to bed.

4. Give an insulin injection if your diabetes care team instructs you to do so (dose, if ordered = _____).

5. Eat a bedtime snack. This may not always be needed in the future, but the insulin dose is still being adjusted. Some ideas for this snack include: cereal and milk, toast and peanut butter, a slice of pizza, yogurt and graham crackers, or cheese and crackers.

E. *The next morning:*

1. Check the blood sugar and the urine ketones upon awakening (if blood sugar is less than 70 mg/dL [3.9 mmol/L], drink 4–6 oz of juice promptly).

2. If your physician has instructed you to give the morning insulin at home, then follow your insulin dosing plan (see Table). Follow the steps listed above (see letter "C") for last night's meal dose if you have questions.

3. If you have been instructed to wait to give the morning dose until after coming to the clinic, check the blood sugar and the urine ketones upon awakening (if blood sugar is less than 70 mg/dL [3.9 mmol/L], drink 4-6 oz of juice promptly).

4. If you are coming/returning to the clinic the next day, you may be asked to do any of the options below:
   □ Take your insulin shot at home (as above) and eat breakfast before coming.
   □ Eat breakfast at home, and then come to the clinic for your insulin injection.
   □ Bring your breakfast to the clinic, and eat it after the insulin has been given.
   □ Bring all blood checking supplies and materials you received the first day back to the clinic (including your log book, Pink Panther book, insulin and supplies).

Table

Insulin Injection Dosing – Onset Day 2*						
	Blood/ CGM Sugar mg/dL (mmol/L)	A.M.	Lunch	P.M.	Dinner	Bedtime
A) Long-Acting Insulin _____						
B) Intermediate-Acting Insulin (NPH) _____						
C) Rapid-Acting Insulin (sliding scale) _____	70-150 (3.9-8.3)					
	150-250 (8.3-13.9)					
Above 300 mg/dL or 16.7 mmol/L, call diabetes care-provider after ketones checked.	250-350 (13.9-19.4)					
	350-450 (19.4-25.0)					
	>450 (2.5)					

* This Table will be filled out by your diabetes care-provider as he or she has instructed.

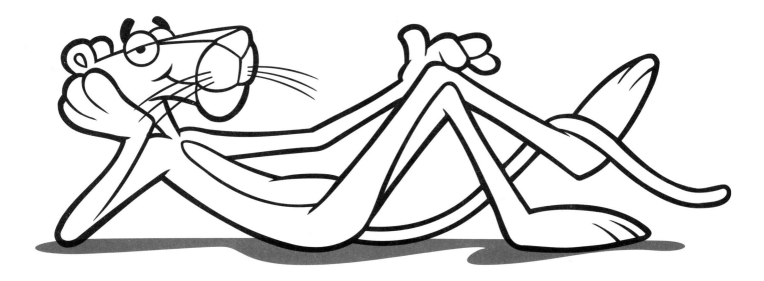

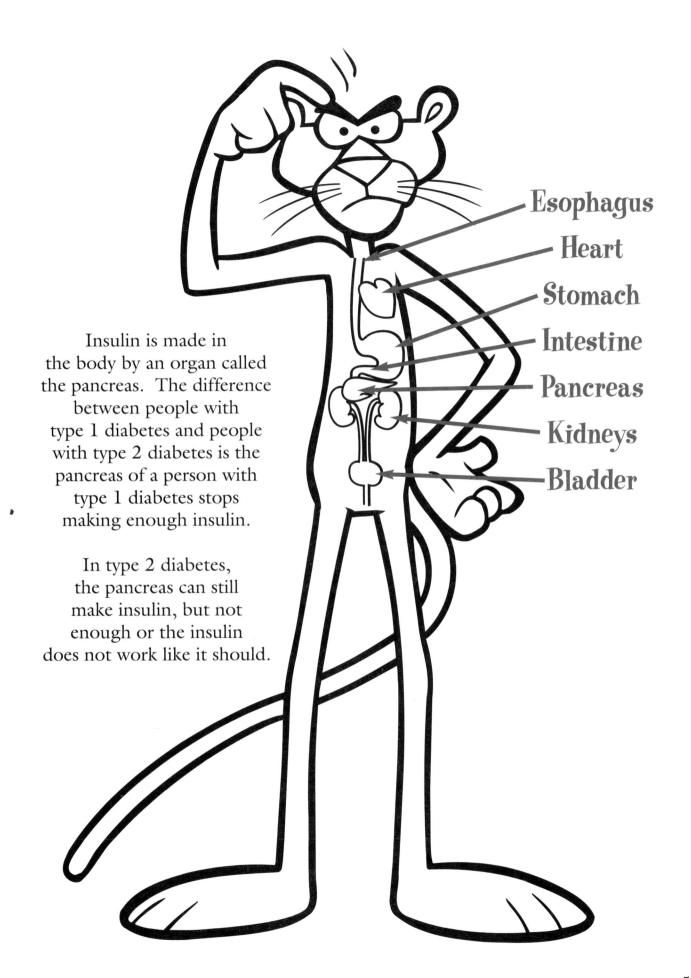

Insulin is made in the body by an organ called the pancreas. The difference between people with type 1 diabetes and people with type 2 diabetes is the pancreas of a person with type 1 diabetes stops making enough insulin.

In type 2 diabetes, the pancreas can still make insulin, but not enough or the insulin does not work like it should.

Esophagus

Heart

Stomach

Intestine

Pancreas

Kidneys

Bladder

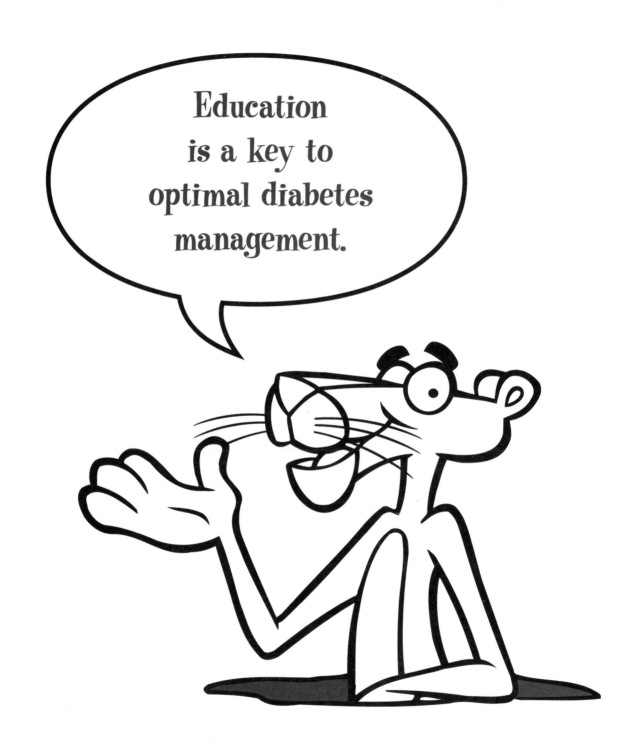

Chapter 1 – The Importance of Education in Diabetes

Chapter 2

What is Diabetes?

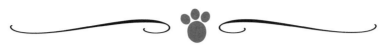

Type 1 diabetes (Childhood, Juvenile, Insulin-dependent) is due to not enough insulin being made in the pancreas (see picture and Chapter 3). The most common signs are:

• **frequent passing of urine (polyuria)**

• **constant thirst (polydipsia)**

• **weight loss**

For people with type 1 diabetes, insulin must be taken by injection. Insulin cannot be taken as a pill, because the stomach acid would destroy it.

Type 2 diabetes (Adult-onset, or Non-insulin dependent diabetes) is different from type 1 diabetes (see Chapter 4). Although the above symptoms may be present, there are often no symptoms at diagnosis. A diagnosis can be made using plasma glucose values or a HbA1c value (see Table). Insulin is still made, but not enough, or it doesn't work very well. People with type 2 diabetes can sometimes use pills (which are not insulin) and diet and exercise to control their diabetes (see Chapter 4). Eating healthy food and exercising are also important for people with type 1 diabetes, but they will always need to take insulin shots.

Insulin allows sugar to pass into our cells to be used for energy. It also turns off the body's making of sugar. When not enough insulin is present, the sugar cannot pass into the body's cells. The sugar is high in the blood and it passes out in the urine. Frequent passing of urine is the result. (See Figures on the next 2 pages.) A goal of treatment is to give insulin back to the person as needed to replace the insulin they are unable to make.

Because sugar cannot be used for energy without insulin, the body breaks down fat for energy. **Ketones** are the result of using fat for energy.

When insulin treatment begins, the urine/blood ketones gradually disappear (see Chapter 5). After a few days, the blood sugars come into range and the excess passing of urine and drinking of water will decrease. Weight is gained back, the appetite normalizes and the person starts to feel much better.

Pre-diabetes refers to the period before developing diabetes. It is usually detected in people who will develop type 1 diabetes because they have had the blood test to detect islet cell antibodies (see Chapters 3 and 32). Pre-type 2 diabetes is very common. It is usually diagnosed in people who are overweight and who have borderline blood sugar and/or HbA1c levels (see Chapter 14). Weight loss and exercise can help delay or prevent the onset of type 2 diabetes (but not type 1 diabetes).

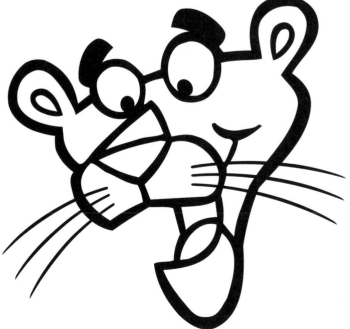

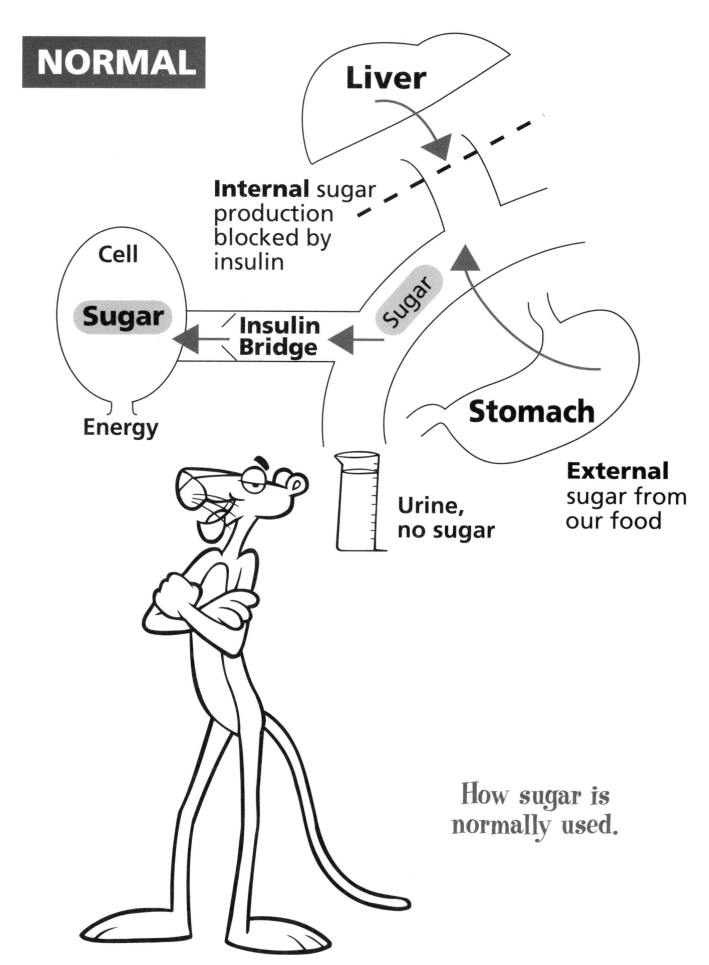

NORMAL

Liver

Internal sugar production blocked by insulin

Cell

Sugar

Energy

Insulin Bridge

Sugar

Stomach

Urine, no sugar

External sugar from our food

How sugar is normally used.

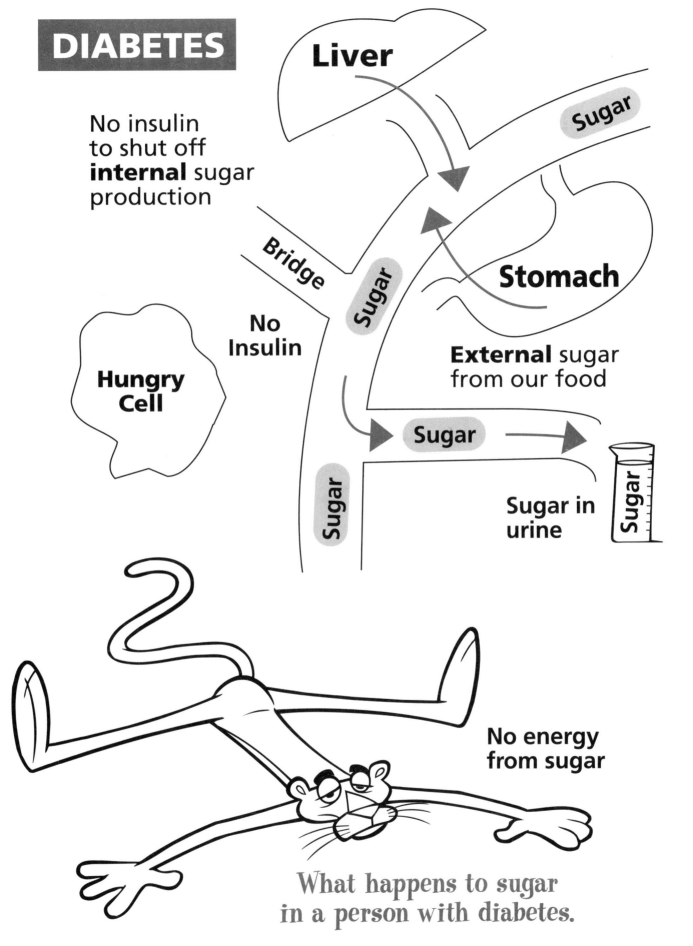

DIABETES

Liver

No insulin to shut off **internal** sugar production

Sugar

Bridge

Sugar

No Insulin

Stomach

Hungry Cell

External sugar from our food

Sugar

Sugar

Sugar in urine

Sugar

No energy from sugar

What happens to sugar in a person with diabetes.

Table

Diagnostic Criteria for Diabetes		
Hemoglobin A1c	Blood/CGM Glucost: mg/dL (mmol/L)	
HbA1c: % (mmol/mol)*	Fasting/ Before Meals*	Bedtime/Overnight
Normal (Non-Diabetic) <6.0% (<42)	70-100 (3.9-5.5)	70-140 (3.9-7.8)
Borderline Levels 5.7-6.4% (39-46)	100-125 (5.5-6.9)	140-200 (7.8-11.1)
Diabetes >6.4% (>46)	>125 (6.9)	>200 (11.1)

< = less than; > = greater than

† After heavy exercise, a goal of 130-150 (7.2-8.3) might be a safer level at bedtime.

* Values in parentheses represent mmol/L (glucose) or mmol/mol (HbA1c). The HbA1c levels are as recommended by the ADA in 2014.

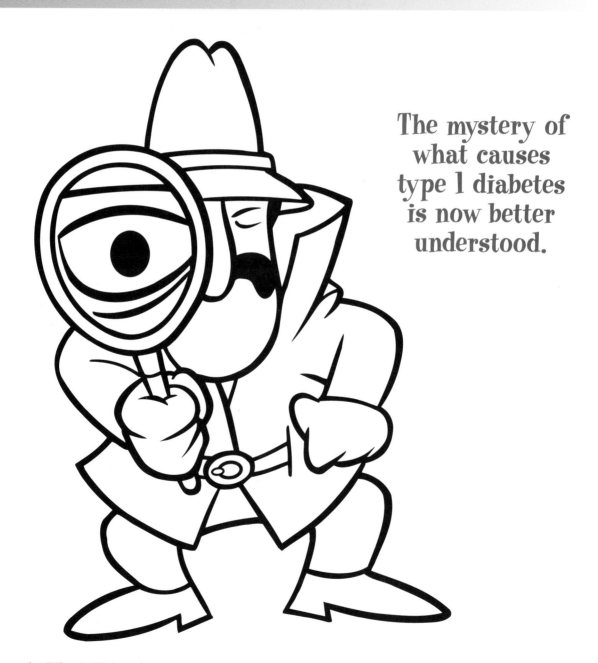

The mystery of what causes type 1 diabetes is now better understood.

Chapter 3
Type 1 Diabetes

WHAT CAUSES DIABETES?

Type 1 diabetes is believed to be caused by three things: genetics, self-allergy and possibly a virus (or other stimulant).

GENETICS (INHERITANCE)

Genes come from both mom and dad and can make someone more likely to get diabetes. Over half of the people who get type 1 diabetes have inherited the gene combination DR3/DR4 (one is from mom and one is from dad).

SELF-ALLERGY (AUTOIMMUNITY)

* The immune system protects the body from possible harm, such as from an infection.
* An allergy is a reaction by the body's immune system to something it thinks doesn't belong inside the body.
* Self-allergy (autoimmunity) is when a person's body develops an allergy against one of its own parts. In this case, the allergy is against the islet ('eye-let') cells in the pancreas where insulin is made. When the islet cells have been damaged, the immune system makes something called antibodies. These antibodies are present in the blood and are markers of the immune system attacking the pancreas.

Antibodies that may be found in the blood of people with type 1 diabetes are:
* IAA (insulin autoantibody)
* GAD antibody
* ICA512 antibody
* ZnT8 antibody
* Islet cell antibodies (by fluorescent stain)

Sometimes these antibodies are present for many years before the signs of diabetes appear. Being able to identify antibodies has allowed studies to try to prevent type 1 diabetes (see Chapter 32 on research).

VIRUS (OR OTHER STIMULANT)

Having a certain gene makeup may allow a virus or other stimulant (currently unknown) to get to the islet cells (where insulin is made) and cause damage. Once the damage has occurred, the self-allergy likely begins.

DIAGNOSIS AND TREATMENT

The **symptoms** of diabetes have been discussed in Chapter 2. The **treatment** of type 1 diabetes is always with insulin (Chapter 8). Frequent blood sugar checking or use of a continuous glucose monitor (Chapters 7 and 29) is important. Following a food plan (Chapter 12) and daily exercise (Chapter 13) are also important.

Often a **"honeymoon"** time begins a few weeks or months after a person with type 1 diabetes starts insulin shots. The insulin dose may go down and it may seem like the person does not have diabetes, but **THEY DO!** This period may last from a few weeks to a few years.

Checking **blood sugars** at least four times per day is essential for people with type 1 diabetes. The eventual use of an insulin pump (Chapter 28) or a continuous glucose monitor (CGM; Chapter 29) may help make diabetes management easier.

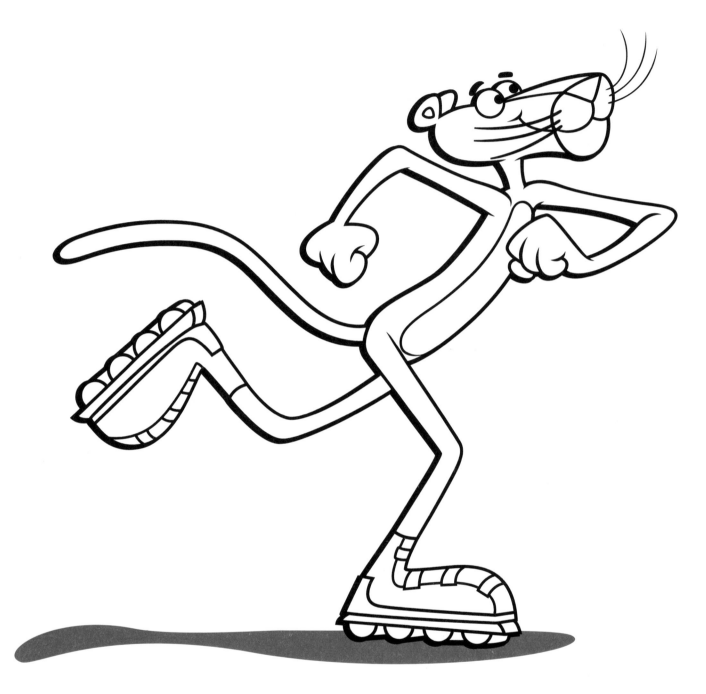

Thirty to sixty minutes of exercise
at least five times a week is important
for people with diabetes.

Chapter 4
Type 2 Diabetes

Type 2 diabetes (previously referred to as Adult-onset diabetes or Non-insulin dependent diabetes) is the most common type to occur in adults over age 40 years. It is also becoming more common in youth (particularly in overweight teenagers). Native-American, African-American and Latino youth have an increased risk for type 2 diabetes.

CAUSES

Type 2 diabetes is partly inherited (genetic). It is also linked with being overweight and not getting enough exercise. It is often called a "disease of life-styles." Our ancestors were very active and ate less. We now live in a world of automobile travel, television, computers, video games, and high calorie fast foods.

Type 2 (Adult-onset) diabetes does not occur as a result of the self-allergy like type 1 diabetes. Therefore, the antibodies (found in type 1 diabetes) are not present in the blood. Type 2 diabetes is often associated with being overweight.

People with type 2 diabetes initially may have normal or high insulin levels. Being overweight leads to "insulin resistance." The insulin just does not work well. In contrast, people with type 1 diabetes have low or no insulin. The two conditions are both called diabetes. Both result in high sugar levels, but the causes are VERY different from each other.

SYMPTOMS

The symptoms can be the same as with type 1 diabetes (Chapter 2). They may be:

- Frequent drinking of liquids
- Frequent urination (going to the bathroom)
- Infections
- Sores that heal slowly
- No energy

Many people don't have any symptoms. These people are sometimes diagnosed by a high blood sugar that is measured on a routine physical exam or with an elevated hemoglobin A1c (HbA1c) level (see Chapter 14). Others are diagnosed when they have a high blood sugar level during an Oral Glucose Tolerance Test (see *"Understanding Diabetes,"* Chapter 4).

TREATMENT: CHANGES IN LIFESTYLE ARE VERY IMPORTANT.

- Eating foods with fewer calories and carbohydrates as well as less fat is very important.

- Getting at least 60 minutes of exercise five to seven days a week is important.

- Checking blood sugars (like people with type 1 diabetes) is helpful (Chapter 7). The blood sugar values can tell how well the person is doing.

- The HbA1c level reflects how high blood sugar levels have been over the previous three months and should be measured every three months (see Chapter 14). The level reflects the likelihood of later diabetes complications (Chapter 23).

- If at diagnosis a person has ketones, or very high blood sugar or HbA1c values, insulin shots are usually needed. The shots may also be needed during times of illness.

- Medications by mouth can be tried if the blood sugar and HbA1c levels return to near normal (Chapter 14). Often, by losing weight and exercising, blood sugar levels do return to near normal.

- The medicines taken by mouth ARE NOT insulin. When taken, these medicines may cause the pancreas to make more insulin. They can also make the body more sensitive to its own insulin. Some medicines also cause the liver to release less sugar into the blood.

- One of these medicines is called **metformin (Glucophage®).**

  - This medicine is usually tried first.

  - Rarely, it can cause an upset stomach. Starting with lower doses and gradually increasing the dose often helps.

- If a person becomes sick, this medicine should be stopped until they are well. Blood sugars and urine ketones should be checked. Insulin shots may be needed during the illness. Call your doctor or nurse if you are not sure what to do.

- There are other medicines taken by mouth that can be tried if metformin isn't working well.

- We are learning more about type 2 diabetes in adolescents from a current study. Over a period of three years, half of the patients in the study needed insulin in order to control their blood sugar levels.

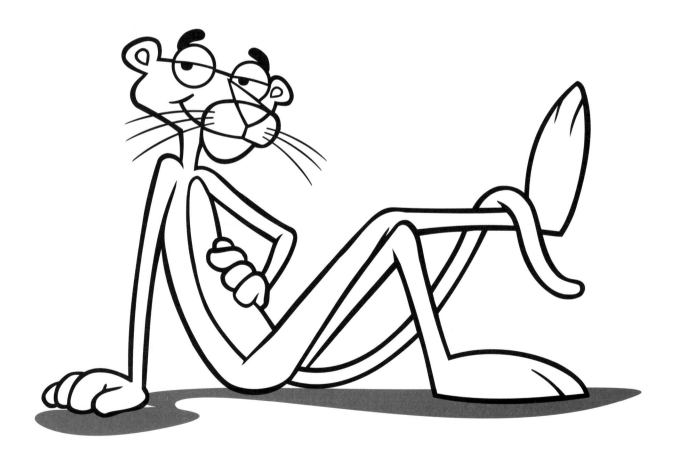

Chapter 5
Checking Ketones

Checking ketones is very easy and very important.

A. FOR A NEWLY DIAGNOSED PERSON

The first goal for new patients is to clear their ketones.

Ketones come from fat breakdown. Insulin stops fat breakdown and prevents ketones from being made.

A second goal is to lower blood sugar levels.

Insulin also turns off sugar production from the liver and allows sugar to enter the body's cells (see Figures in Chapter 2).

B. FOR A PERSON WITH KNOWN DIABETES

When to check for ketones (either in urine or blood):

• During any illness

• With a very high blood/CGM sugar (e.g., above 300 mg/dL [>16.7 mmol/L])

• If an insulin shot is missed

• After vomiting even once

• With a blockage of an insulin pump catheter or pump failure

If ketones are present, extra insulin can be given to stop the ketones from being made. (Ketones need to be detected early and extra insulin given or the person may get very sick; see Chapter 15 on diabetic ketoacidosis [DKA].)

C. HOW TO CHECK FOR KETONES

A method to check for ketones must always be in the home and taken along on trips. Checking ketones and giving extra insulin can help prevent the person from becoming very sick. Ketones can be checked using either urine or a drop of blood. The urine strips are cheaper, although the blood has the advantage of telling how high the ketones are at that moment. Some people do the urine ketone check first, and only do the blood ketones if the urine shows moderate or large ketones.

URINE KETONES

The two main strips used are:

1. Ketostix®: This strip is dipped into the urine and is read as negative, trace, small, moderate, large, or extra large after *exactly* 15 seconds.

2. Chemstrip K®: This strip is dipped into the urine and is read as negative, trace, small, moderate, large or extra large after *exactly* 60 seconds.

   All urine ketones strips (including Ketostix) must be thrown out six months after the bottle is opened.

BLOOD KETONES

Some people prefer to use a meter to check blood ketones. There are now several meters for checking blood ketone levels. These include the Precision Xtra® (Abbott labs) and the Nova Max® ketone meter (Nova® Biomedical).

For the Precision Xtra, the method is as follows:

• The blood ketone strip is inserted with the three black bars going into the meter.

• Then a drop of blood is placed on the white target area at the end of the strip.

• The result is given in 10 seconds.

Table

Comparison of Blood and Urine Ketone Readings

Blood Ketone (mmol/L)	Strip color	Urine Ketone Level	Action to take
less than 0.6	slight/no color change	negative	normal - no action needed
0.6 to 1.0	light purple	small to moderate	extra insulin & fluids**
1.1 to 3.0	dark purple	moderate to large*	call MD or RN**
greater than 3.0	very dark purple	very large*	go directly to the E.R.

*It is usually advised to call a healthcare-provider for a blood ketone level greater than 1.0 or with urine ketone readings of moderate or large.

**If the blood glucose level is below 150 mg/dL (<8.3 mmol/L), a liquid with sugar (e.g., juice) should be taken so more insulin can be safely given.

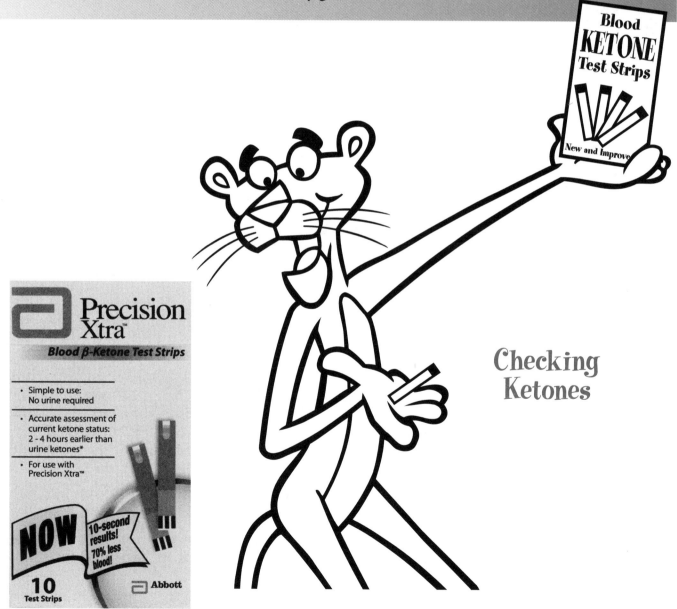

Checking Ketones

Chapter 6
Low Blood Sugar
(Hypoglycemia or Insulin Reaction)

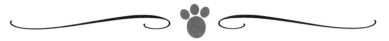

Anyone who has been given insulin can have low blood sugar (hypoglycemia or a "reaction"). Blood sugars below 70 mg/dL (3.9 mmol/L) are considered low and are usually related to the person having one or more of the signs outlined below. **A "true low" blood sugar is a value less than 60 mg/dL (3.3 mmol/L) which is a level not likely to occur in people who do not have diabetes or another disorder.** (The term blood/CGM glucose level indicates that the value may be from a finger stick or a continuous glucose monitor [CGM]. The terms "sugar" and "glucose" are used interchangeably in this book.)

MAIN CAUSES OF LOW BLOOD/CGM SUGAR:

- Extra exercise (the low may be "delayed," occurring during the night)

- Too much insulin/wrong dose

- Taking bath, shower or hot tub too soon after injection (dangerous)

- A previous low blood/CGM sugar during the day ("hypoglycemia can cause further hypoglycemia")

- Illness, especially with vomiting

- Late or missed meals or snacks

- Alcohol intake

FREQUENT SIGNS OF A LOW BLOOD SUGAR:

- Hunger

- Feeling shaky, sweaty and/or weak

- Confusion

- Sleepiness (at unusual times)

- Changes in behavior or mood (for example: cranky, arguing, unreasonable)

- Double vision

- The signs of nighttime lows may be the same, or may include waking up alert, crying, or having bad dreams

Low blood sugar can come on quickly. It must be treated immediately by the person (if able) or by someone who is nearby at the time. A person with a low blood sugar should not be left alone until the blood sugar has returned to normal.

The **"rule of 15"** is to take 15 grams of rapid-acting carbohydrate (e.g., four dextrose tablets) and to **recheck the blood sugar level in 15 minutes.** If lows are not treated, eventual loss of consciousness or a seizure may occur. It is important not to over-treat lows. While someone with a low will often be very hungry, overtreatment can cause a rebound high blood sugar. Use finger-stick blood sugar levels in follow-up as the CGM values are delayed by 10 minutes and may result in excessive treatment Different levels of reactions (mild, moderate, severe) and treatment for each level are discussed below and in the table in this chapter.

MILD, MODERATE AND SEVERE LOW BLOOD SUGAR

With a "MILD" low blood sugar (also see Table), the following apply:

- Give sugar (best in liquid form) such as four ounces of juice or sugary drink (soda, pop, etc.). Dextrose tablets (four) work well.

- When possible, a blood/CGM sugar level should be checked.

- It takes 10 to 20 minutes for the blood sugar to rise after treatment.

- Re-check the blood/CGM sugar level after 15 minutes to make sure the level is above 70 mg/dL (3.9 mmol/L).

- If it is still below this level, the liquid sugar or Dextrose tablets should be given again. Follow the steps above.

- Wait another 15 minutes to recheck the blood/CGM sugar level.

- If the blood/CGM sugar level is above 70 mg/dL (3.9 mmol/L), consider giving solid food. The reason for waiting to give the solid food is that it may soak up the liquid sugar and slow the time for the sugar to get into the blood.

- The person should not return to activity until the blood sugar is above 70 mg/dL (3.9 mmol/L).

- If the low is at bedtime, it is important to recheck the blood/CGM sugar, as above, and again during the night to make sure the level stays up.

- If a low blood sugar occurs when it is time for an insulin shot, always treat the low first. Make sure the blood/CGM sugar level is above 70 mg/dL (3.9 mmol/L) before giving the shot.

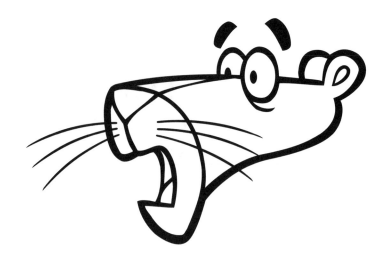

With a "MODERATE" reaction (also see Table), the following apply:

- Put half a tube of Insta-Glucose® or cake gel between the gums and cheeks. Rub the cheeks and stroke the throat to help with swallowing.

- If a person has a low blood sugar and can't keep food down or has difficulty getting the blood/CGM level up, low-dose glucagon, one unit per year of age up to 15 units, can be given under the skin just like insulin - with an insulin syringe. The dose can be repeated every 20 minutes until the blood sugar is up. Once glucagon is mixed, it usually can continue to be used for about 24 hours before it gels. Intranasal-glucagon can be used instead of the injection. If the person has not responded to two doses of glucagon, emergency help may be needed.

With a "SEVERE" reaction (also see Table), the following apply:

- If a seizure or complete loss of consciousness occurs, it is usually necessary to give a shot of glucagon or to use intranasal-glucagon.

- If no response in 15-20 minutes, may need to call 911.

- If on an insulin pump, remember to disconnect or suspend the insulin delivery.

- Your doctor or nurse should be called prior to the next insulin shot, as the amount of insulin you give may need to be changed.

Glucagon

Glucagon Injection

- Glucagon injection will make the blood sugar rise, usually in 10 to 20 minutes. Although the result of giving glucagon is the opposite of giving insulin, it is <u>NOT</u> sugar.

- After mixing, glucagon can be given with an insulin syringe, just like insulin.

The amount of injected glucagon to give varies with age:

- Under 6 years: can be given a full 30 unit syringe (0.3 cc).

- 6-12 years: can be given a full 50 unit syringe (0.5 cc).

- Over 12 years: can be given a full 100 unit syringe (1.0 cc).

- If the person does not respond within 15 to 20 minutes, the paramedics (911) should be called.

- Instructions are simplified in the school setting (Chapter 25), with instructions to give 0.5 cc if <16 years old or 1.0 cc if ≥16 years old. It is important just to get glucagon in.

- Glucagon should always be readily available and taken on trips. It will spoil if it freezes or gets above 90°F (32°C). Intranasal-glucagon is now an alternative (see below).

Intranasal-glucagon

The availability of intranasal-glucagon will make the treatment of moderate to severe hypoglycemia much easier. This is particularly true for the school or work setting, where a nurse or trained family member may not be available. Severe lows can occur rapidly during the day, with altered eating, exercise or insulin boluses. In contrast, they usually occur at night only if the glucose level has been below 60 mg/dL (3.3 mmol/L) for over two hours.

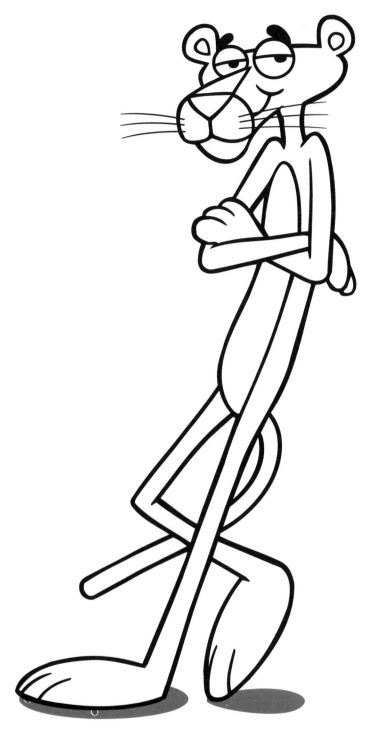

The plastic device for administration of the intranasal-glucagon requires only one step for administration, the depression of the plunger. It raises the blood sugar to above 70 mg/dL (3.9 mmol/L) in an average of 16 minutes (compared to 13 minutes for intramuscular-glucagon). This difference is inconsequential. The intranasal-glucagon has been shown to still be effective with nasal congestion. It may be easier to carry outside of the home than the injectable glucagon.

Table

Hypoglycemia: Treatment of Low Blood Sugar (B.S.) When Possible Always Check Blood Sugar Level!

(Note, during recovery from hypoglycemia, we prefer use of blood sugar sticks rather than using CGM values, which may be 10 minutes behind.)

LEVEL	MILD	MODERADO	SEVERO
Alertness	ALERT	NOT ALERT **Unable to drink safely (choking risk)** Needs help from another person	UNRESPONSIVE **Loss of consciousness** **Seizure** **Needs constant adult help (position of safety)** *Give nothing by mouth (extreme choking risk)*
Simptoms	Mood Changes Shaky, Sweaty Hungry Fatigue, Weak Pale	Lack of Focus Headache Confused Disoriented 'Out of Control' (bite, kick) *Can't* Self-treat	Loss of Consciousness Seizure
Actions to take	• Check B.S. • Give 2-8 oz sugary fluid (amount age dependent) • Recheck B.S. in 10-15 min. • B.S. *<70 mg/dL (<3.9 mmol/L), repeat sugary fluid and recheck in 10-20 min. • B.S. *>70 mg/dL (>3.9 mmol/L), (give a solid snack) • Slight risk for more lows in next 24 hours (after any low blood sugar)	• *Place in position of safety* • Check B.S. • If on insulin pump, may disconnect or suspend until fully recovered from low blood sugar **(awake and alert)** • Give Insta-Glucose or cake decorating gel – put between gums and cheek and rub in. Can use intranasal-glucagon if needed. • Look for person to 'wake up' • Recheck B.S. in 10-20 min. • *Once alert* – follow "actions" under 'Mild' column • Moderate risk for more lows in next 24 hours	• *Place in position of safety* • Check B.S. • If on insulin pump, disconnect or suspend until fully recovered from low blood sugar **(awake and alert)** • Glucagon: *can be given with an insulin syringe* like insulin: • Under 6 years: **30 units (3/10 cc)** • 6-12 years: **50 units (1/2 cc)** • Over 12 years: **100 units (all of dose or 1 cc)** • If giving 50 or 100 unit doses, may use syringe in box and inject through clothing • Can use intranasal-glucagon instead of injection. • **Check B.S. every 10-15 min. until *>70 mg/dL (>3.9 mmol/L)** • <u>**If no response, may need to call 911**</u> • **Check B.S. every hour for 4-5 hours** • High risk for more lows for 24 hours (need to increase food intake and decrease insulin doses)
Recovery time	10-20 minutes	20-45 minutes	**Call RN/MD** and report the episode. Effects can last 2-12 hours

*< sign means "less than" — > sign means "greater than"

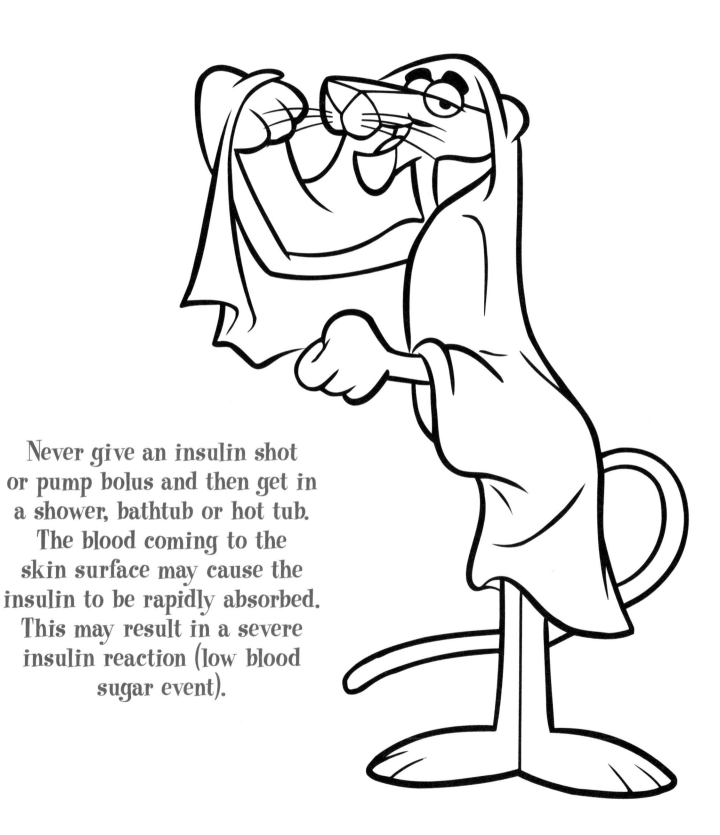

Never give an insulin shot
or pump bolus and then get in
a shower, bathtub or hot tub.
The blood coming to the
skin surface may cause the
insulin to be rapidly absorbed.
This may result in a severe
insulin reaction (low blood
sugar event).

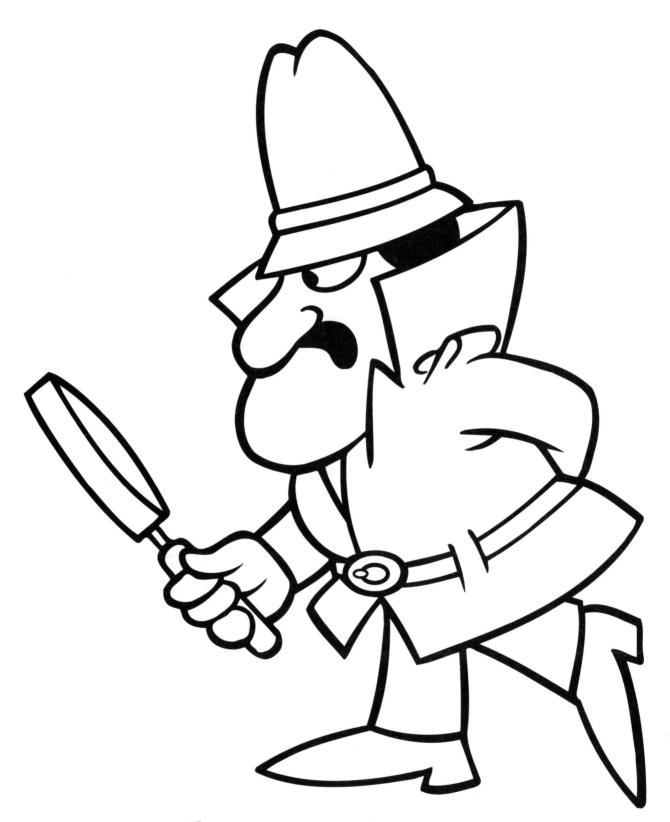

It is important for adults to
keep an eye on younger children
for **signs** of **low sugar.**

Chapter 6 – Low Blood Sugar (Hypoglycemia or Insulin Reaction)

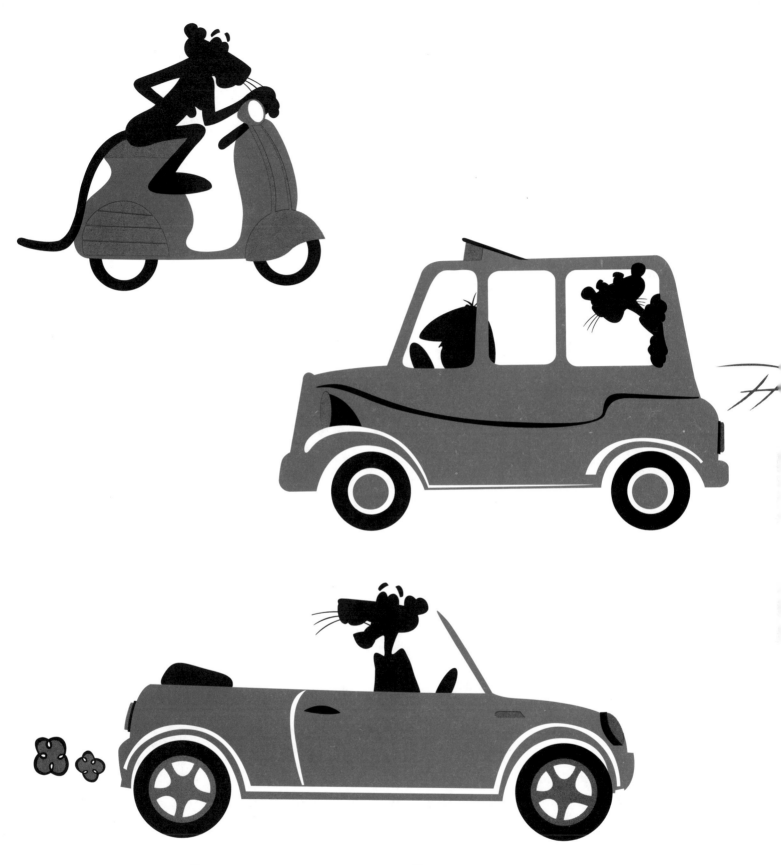

It is important to <u>always</u> check
a blood/CGM sugar before driving.

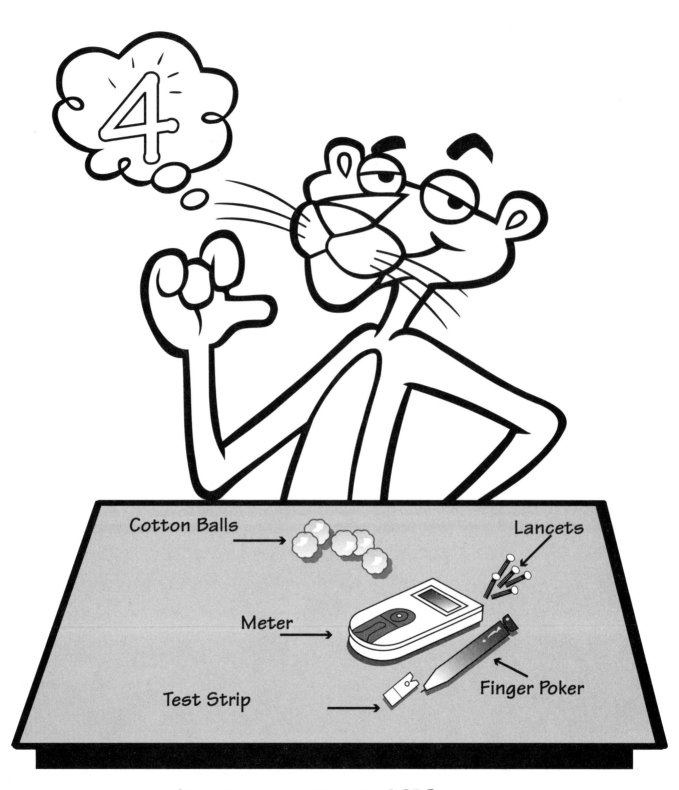

Check your blood/CGM sugars
(four or more times each day), including
before eating, exercising and going to bed.

Chapter 7
Blood/CGM Sugar (Glucose) Monitoring

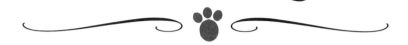

The FDA has approved the use of the Dexcom G5 and G6 and the FreeStyle Libre Flash continuous glucose monitors (CGM) for deciding on insulin dosages (see Chapter 29 on CGM). Similarly, the FDA approved the MiniMed/Medtronic 670G artificial pancreas system in which the insulin pump delivers insulin based on CGM glucose levels. However, fingerstick blood sugars must still be done, even if using a CGM. Some CGMs must be calibrated twice daily using fingerstick values. Also, most physicians recommend checking a fingerstick blood sugar with hypoglycemic episodes or anytime the CGM value is out of range (e.g., above 250 (13.9) or below 70 mg/dL (3.9 mmol/L). This is done for verification. It is important to remember that some CGM readings may not be accurate if the person has recently received a medicine containing acetaminophen (e.g., Tylenol). This is not a problem with the Dexcom G6 or Libre Flash. In summary, blood sugar checking is still important, and is the major emphasis of this chapter.

Blood sugar checking involves obtaining a small sample of blood using a small lancing device ("poker"). A small drop of blood is placed on a disposable test strip. A meter is then used to calculate the sugar level in the sample. The blood sample is usually taken from a fingertip. Some people use an "alternate site," such as the forearm (see below).

IF NOT USING A CGM, BLOOD SUGARS SHOULD BE CHECKED:

- Four or more times each day (usually before meals and exercise and before bedtime)
- Several times each week, approximately two hours after each meal, to assess the adequacy of the meal insulin dose
- Anytime the symptoms of a low blood sugar are felt (see Table 1 and Chapter 6)
- Occasionally during the night
- Anytime unusual symptoms occur (e.g., frequent voiding)

IF USING A CGM, CHECK BLOOD SUGARS:

- With high or low CGM values (see above)
- Anytime the person has a hypoglycemic episode
- If the person has taken acetaminophen (e.g. Tylenol)

GOALS (Similar for fingerstick and CGM glucose values)

The target blood/CGM sugar values are different for each age group and are shown in the Table 1. At least half of the blood/CGM sugar values at each time of day should be in the desired range for age. The blood/CGM sugar ranges are shown for both before meals/fasting and for bedtime/overnight.

Table 1: Blood/CGM Sugar Levels

NON-DIABETIC NORMAL VALUES*

Normal (fasting)**	70-100 (3.9-5.5)
Normal (random)	70-140 (3.9-7.8)

GOALS FOR PEOPLE WITH DIABETES*

Diabetes management recommendations always need to be tailored to the individual. Higher targets may be considered if: history of hypoglycemic unawareness/severe hypoglycemia, use of NPH at bedtime, poor access to testing strips or CGM, very low insulin requirements, athletes and infants or toddlers. In young children, use of CGM and insulin pumps may be necessary to reach goals safely.

	Before Meals Fasting	Bedtime Overnight
0-5 years	70-150 (3.9-8.3)	100-180*** (5.5-10.0)
6-17 years	70-130 (3.9-7.2)	90-150*** (5.0-8.3)
18 years and up	70-130 (3.9-7.2)	90-150*** (5.0-8.3)

Low Values*		Possible Symptoms
Low	Below 70 (Below 3.9)	Sweating Hunger Shakiness
"True low"	Below 60 (Below 3.3)	Confusion. If not treated, can lead to seizure or unconsciousness episode

High Values*		Possible Symptoms
High	200-400 (11.1-22.2)	Low energy Frequent urination
Very high	400-800 (22.2-44.4)	Stomachache Rapid breathing If not treated, can lead to DKA

Remember to check ketones if > 300 mg / dL (16.7 mmol/L)

*Blood/CGM glucose levels in mg/dL (mmol/L)

**Most values for non-diabetic children are in this range. However, occasional values down to 60 mg/dL (3.3 mmol/L) are still normal.

***If a very heavy exercise day, 130 mg/dL (7.3 mmol/L) might be a better lower level.

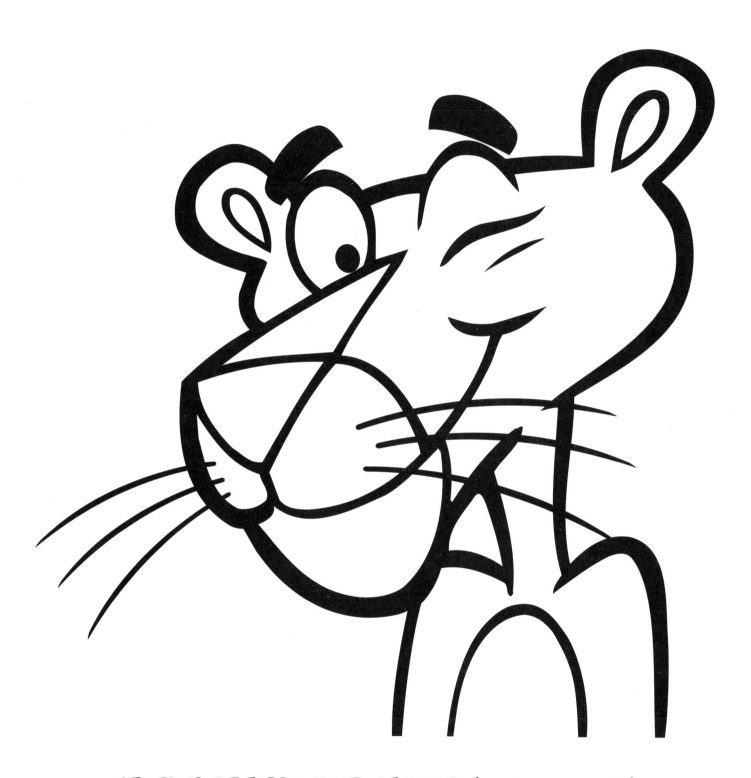

ALWAYS BRING YOUR METER (and log book) TO YOUR CLINIC VISITS.

DOING THE BLOOD SUGARS

Finger-Pokes

How to do the blood sugar

- Get poker ready; insert lancet (change daily).

- Wash hands with soap and warm water; dry. Traces of sugar on the fingertip can greatly raise the value.

- Poke side or tip (not ball) of chosen finger or of arm (alternate site values).

- To get enough blood, hold hand down (below heart level) and "milk" the finger.

- Put the drop of blood on the blood sugar strip as taught for each meter.

- Hold cotton ball on poke site to stop bleeding.

METERS

We do not recommend one meter over another. However, some cheap, low-quality meters are now being sold in stores. If uncertain, check with your diabetes care-provider.

- We like meters that can store at least the last 100 values.

- The meter must also be able to be downloaded by the family or clinic.

- Strips requiring smaller amounts of blood make it easier for young children.

- Make sure the code in the meter matches the code for the strips (if required).

- **The meter must always be brought to the clinic visit.**

The Roche company has developed a meter, the ACCU-CHEK® Aviva Connect, which includes an app which allows bluetooth transmission of fingerstick blood sugar values to a smart phone or other mobile device. The lancing device has a comfort dial which can be adjusted for the desired depth to obtain in the drop of blood. The lancing device contains 6 lancets for easing switching of lancets. It also has an app which can be set up when the family is ready to use the blood sugar measurement to help calculate an insulin bolus dose to give. This insulin dose calculation is similar to what insulin pumps do, but it is for people giving insulin injections. The grams of carbs to be eaten are entered into the meter. Data for insulin to carb ratios and the correction (sensitivity) factor are pre-programmed into the meter for the individual patient for different times of the day. The meter also subtracts active insulin ("insulin on board") from recently administered insulin (if entered into meter). This insulin-dose calculator will be particularly helpful when young children do not have their parents available to determine dose calculations.

ALTERNATE SITE CHECKING

Some meters require such a small drop of blood that it can be obtained from the arm or another site. However, if feeling low, the fingertip must be used as circulation is not as good in other sites and the true blood sugar level may be delayed by 10-20 minutes.

LOG BOOKS

It is important to record meter results or to download meters at regular intervals.

- Look for patterns of highs and lows.

- If too many lows occur, insulin dose reductions may be needed (e.g., more than two values per week below 60 mg/dL [3.3 mmol/L]). Results can be sent to the nurse or doctor by fax, email or cloud if help with insulin dose adjustments is needed.

- If too many highs occur, insulin dose increases may be needed (e.g., more than two values at the same time of day in a week above 300 mg/dL [16.7 mmol/L]). Results can be sent to the nurse or doctor by fax, email or cloud if help with insulin dose adjustments is needed (see Table 2: Daily Record Sheet).

- We encourage families to learn to make adjustments. If you send sugar results, you should suggest solutions to your questions, which can be discussed with a doctor or nurse.

- Parents (even of teens) must do or supervise the recording of the values and the sending of the results.

- **Bring the meter and log book to the clinic visit.**

FEELINGS

It is important not to be upset if highs or lows are found. This can make following sugar levels a negative experience. Just use the data to adjust the insulin and/or to prevent future highs or lows. We emphasize that sugars are "in target" or "high" or "low," but not "good" or "bad." The only response should be **"Thank you for following your sugar levels."**

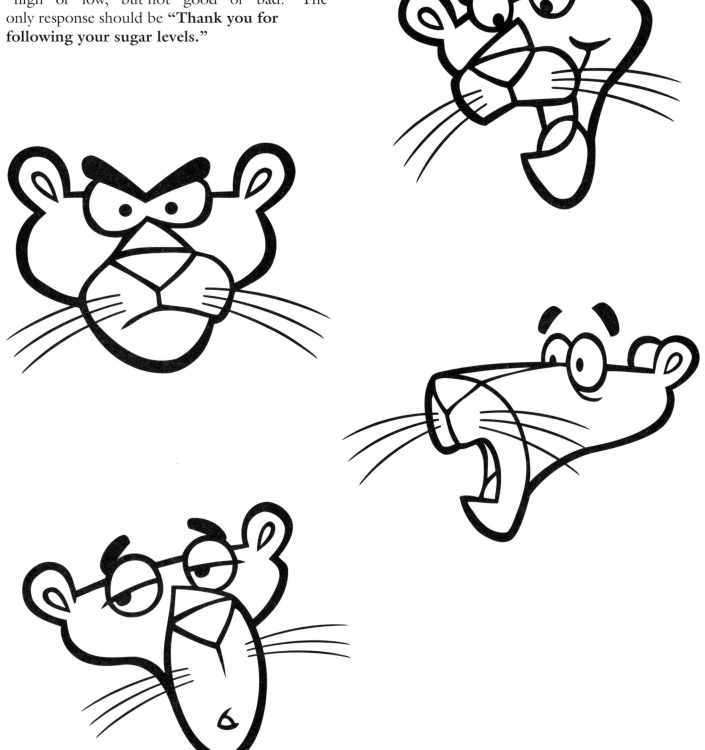

Table 2: Daily Record Sheet

To Nurse Educator: _____

Patient _____ Date of Birth _____

Phone: _____

Physician: _____

Parents: _____

Best time (8 a.m. - 5 p.m.) to reach you: _____

Date		Breakfast Results	Breakfast Insulin Dose	Other (optional) Results	Other (optional) Insulin Dose	Lunch Results	Lunch Insulin Dose	Other (optional) Results	Other (optional) Insulin Dose	Dinner Results	Dinner Insulin Dose	Bedtime Results	Bedtime Insulin Dose	Comments (Exercise, illness, snacks, other)
	Time:													
	BG/Ket:													
	Time:													
	BG/Ket:													
	Time:													
	BG/Ket:													
	Time:													
	BG/Ket:													
	Time:													
	BG/Ket:													
	Time:													
	BG/Ket:													
	Time:													
	BG/Ket:													

Ket = Ketones

Problem Area(s) Noted: _____

Suggested Solution(s): _____

Please note: Make sure insulin doses are included under "Insulin Dose" heading. Copies of this form can be downloaded at http://www.uchs.edu/misc/diabetes/clinschool.html. Download Word or PDF version of Daily Record Sheet (insulin_daily_rec.doc or insulin_daily_rec.pdf).

Chapter 8
Insulin Types and Activity

Insulin is a hormone normally made in the islet ('eye-let') cells of the pancreas. It allows sugar to pass into the body's cells to be used for energy (Chapter 2). It also prevents the liver from making excess sugar and it prevents the breakdown of fat to release ketones into the blood. It is important to understand the type and action of each insulin being used.

WHY ARE INSULIN SHOTS NEEDED?

- Not enough insulin is made in the pancreas of a person with type 1 diabetes.

- Insulin can't be taken as a pill because it would be destroyed by stomach acid.

- People with type 2 diabetes who have ketones or very high blood sugars or HbA1c levels usually take insulin shots, at least in the beginning of treatment.

THERE ARE FOUR TYPES OF INSULIN:

1) *"rapid-acting/short lasting"* (Humalog [Admelog], NovoLog and Apidra) and Regular

   - Humalog (Admelog), NovoLog and Apidra are more rapid-acting than Regular; they peak earlier and do not last as long as Regular insulin.

   - Humalog (Admelog), NovoLog, Apidra and Regular insulins are clear.

   - Humalog (Admelog), NovoLog and Apidra peak in activity about 90 minutes after being given and last 3-4 hours.

2) *"intermediate-lasting"* (NPH)

   - NPH insulin is cloudy and must be mixed prior to drawing from vial.

- The bottles should be turned gently up and down 20 times before drawing the insulin into the syringe.

- NPH insulin peaks 3-8 hours after being given and lasts 12-15 hours.

3) *"long-lasting"* (Lantus® [Basaglar], Levemir®)

   - These are basal (flat-acting, minimal peak) insulins that last approximately 24 hours.

   - They are clear insulins (don't confuse with rapid-acting insulins, which are also clear).

   - Best given in the bottom (buttocks, seat) to make sure the insulin is given into fat, or into a pinch of fat.

4) *"ultra-long lasting"* (Tresiba® [called Degludec in some countries])

   - This is a basal (flat-acting, minimal peak) insulin. Although used on a daily basis, it lasts for up to three days (72 hours). It is still taken once daily.

   - It has lower day-to-day variability of action and may reduce nighttime low blood sugars.

* *Insulin must be stored so that it does not freeze or get over 90º F (32° C) because it will spoil. Otherwise, the insulin vial being used can be kept at room temperature for 30 days.*

HOW AND WHEN IS INSULIN USED?

Most people with type 1 diabetes take two or more shots of insulin each day. It is common to take a long-lasting insulin once daily, with a rapid-acting insulin given before meals (four shots per day).

RAPID-ACTING INSULIN HUMALOG (ADMELOG), NOVOLOG OR APIDRA)

- Rapid-acting insulins are used to stop the rise of the blood sugar after eating food.

- The rapid-acting insulin (or Regular insulin) can be mixed with NPH insulin to give before breakfast and dinner.

- Most people also take a shot of rapid-acting insulin before lunch and before any snacks (unless taking the snack for low blood sugar).

- Rapid-acting insulin should be taken 20 minutes before the meal. This is because the peak insulin activity occurs 90 minutes after injection. In contrast, blood sugars peak 60 minutes after food intake (Figure 1). If the blood sugar is below 80 mg/dL (4.5 mmol/L), then take the insulin at meal time.

- If Regular insulin is being used, the shot is usually taken 30-45 minutes before meals.

- For toddlers whose appetite may be unpredictable the rapid-acting insulin can be given after the meal. Then the dose can be adjusted to fit the amount of food eaten.

- Rapid-acting insulins are also used to "correct" a blood/CGM glucose level that is too high (see Correction Insulin Dose: Chapter 22).

INTERMEDIATE-ACTING INSULIN (NPH)

- NPH insulin has its main effect in 3 to 8 hours (variable) and lasts 12 to 15 hours. It is usually taken twice daily in a syringe with a rapid-acting insulin (Figure 2).

- NPH insulin taken at dinner or bedtime has a peak during the night so that low blood sugars are more common compared to when a basal (long-acting) insulin is used.

- People who take three shots per day sometimes take their NPH at bedtime rather than at dinner to help it last through the night. It then has a lesser chance of causing low blood sugars during the night.

Figure 1

(Reproduced with permission of <u>Diabetes Technology and Therapeutics</u> 12:173, 2010)

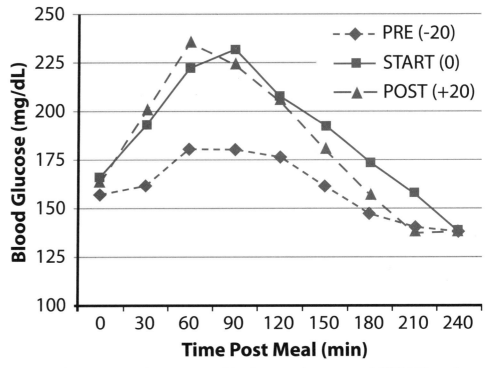

Blood sugar levels when insulin was given 20 minutes prior to a meal ("PRE"), at the beginning of the meal ("START"), or after the meal "POST". The ADA goal for blood sugar at any time after a meal is rto not exceed 180 mg/dL (10mmol/L).

Figure 2

Example of Two Injections a Day Using Rapid Action (or Regular) Insulin and NPH
H=Humalog, NL=NovoLog, AP= Apidra, R=Regular Insulin

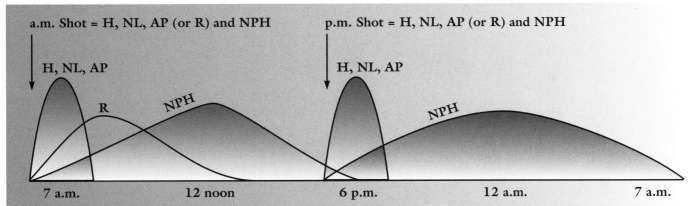

a.m. Shot = H, NL, AP (or R) and NPH   p.m. Shot = H, NL, AP (or R) and NPH

H, NL, AP   R   NPH   H, NL, AP   NPH

7 a.m.   12 noon   6 p.m.   12 a.m.   7 a.m.

Many people receive two injections per day. NPH and a rapid-acting insulin (or Regular) are given prior to breakfast and dinner. When possible, the insulin should be given 20 minutes prior to the meal.

LONG-ACTING INSULINS (LANTUS [BASAGLAR], LEVEMIR OR TRESIBA [Degludec])

Most people using basal-bolus insulin therapy use one of these three insulins for their basal insulin. When using Lantus (Basaglar), Levemir or Tresiba as the basal insulin, the following generally apply (Figures 3):

- The dose is usually taken alone without any other insulin in the syringe (ask your doctor). Then Humalog (Admelog), NovoLog or Apidra are taken 20 minutes before each meal often with an insulin pen (see Figure 3-A).

- Give the insulin into the buttocks (seat) or into a pinch of fat in the stomach (to make sure the insulin is going into the fat).

- The action is very flat and the chance for a low blood sugar is reduced (particularly during the night when the basal insulin is taken in the morning).

- The dose is judged primarily on the morning blood sugar, no matter when the Lantus (Basaglar), Levemir or Tresiba shot is taken. If the fasting blood sugar is consistently above the desired range (Chapter 7) at breakfast, the dose is increased. If below the lower level, the dose is decreased. A consistent time should be chosen to give the Lantus (Basaglar) or Levemir, although the timing of the longer-acting Tresiba can vary from day to day.

- Often Levemir (or Lantus) is given twice a day if it does not seem to last for 24 hours.

- Overnight blood sugar levels (or preferably CGM values) may help to understand the overnight trend.

Figure 3
Use of Lantus (Basaglar), Levemir or Tresiba Insulin

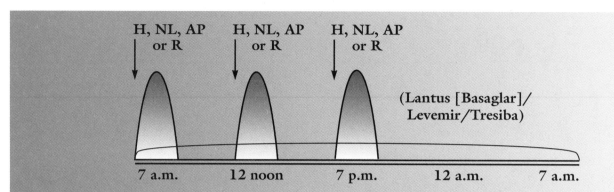

H, NL, AP or R → 7 a.m.

H, NL, AP or R → 12 noon

H, NL, AP or R → 7 p.m.

(Lantus [Basaglar]/ Levemir/Tresiba)

12 a.m. 7 a.m.

In the example in Figure 3, Lantus (Basaglar), Levemir or Tresiba is used as the basal insulin (given in the a.m., or at dinner or at bedtime) and a rapid-acting insulin is taken 20 minutes prior to meals and snacks as described above. This is often referred to as basal-bolus insulin therapy.

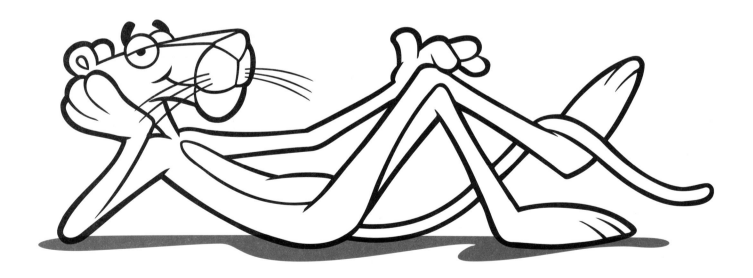

Chapter 9
Drawing Up Insulin and Giving Insulin Injections

The nurse-educator will teach the best way to draw up and to give the insulin. Both are described in this chapter. A section on the use of insulin pens is also included below. Finally, a summary of giving shots to children of different ages is provided.

DRAWING UP INSULIN (Figure 1)

A. Get everything you will need:

- A bottle of each insulin you will use
- Syringe
- Alcohol wipe for tops of bottles
- Log book with current blood sugar results and insulin dose. Please record each blood sugar result and insulin dose in log book.

B. How to draw insulin into the syringe (example of drawing two insulins into a syringe), as with NPH insulin and Regular (or rapid-acting) insulin.

- Know how much of each insulin you need to give (based on "thinking" scales if appropriate – see Chapter 22 in *"Understanding Diabetes"*). Eventually the dose will also be based on carbohydrate counting (Chapter 12) and a correction factor (Chapter 22).
- Wipe off the tops of insulin bottles with alcohol swab.
- Inject air into the intermediate-acting (cloudy) insulin bottle with the bottle sitting upright on the table and remove the needle.*
- Inject air in the clear (rapid-acting) insulin bottle and leave the needle in the bottle.*
- Turn the rapid-acting bottle, with the needle in it, upside down and draw approximately 5 units

of insulin in and out of the syringe to get rid of any air bubbles. (See this chapter in *"Understanding Diabetes"* for specific steps that can be used to get rid of air bubbles.) Draw up the clear rapid-acting insulin you need and remove the needle from the bottle. (Note – if drawing up only one insulin, you have now completed the task. The task would be similar for drawing a long-acting insulin.)

- Mix the cloudy (NPH) insulin by gently turning the bottle up and down 20 times; this mixes the insulin so that it will have a consistent strength.
- Turn the bottle upside down and put the needle into the bottle. Draw up the cloudy insulin into the syringe. *Make sure not to push any rapid-acting insulin already in the syringe back into this bottle.*
- If the insulin bottles have been in the refrigerator, you can warm up the insulin once it is mixed in the syringe by holding the syringe in the closed palm of your hand for a minute. It will be less likely to sting if the insulin is at room temperature.

*An option used by some people is to not put air into the insulin bottles, but to just "vent" the bottles once a week to remove any vacuum. This is done by removing the plunger from the syringe and inserting the needle into the upright insulin bottle. Air will be sucked in through the needle removing the vacuum from the bottle. (The vacuum may otherwise pull insulin from the syringe into the insulin bottle. This is most important if two insulins are being mixed in the same syringe.)

GIVING THE INSULIN

- Choose the area of the body where you are going to give the shot. Use four or more areas and use different sites within the area (see Figure 2).

- Make sure the area where you will be giving the shot is clean.

- Relax the chosen area (see "Different Age Children" section below for techniques).

- Pull up the skin with the finger and thumb (even with short needles).

- Touch the needle to the skin and "punch" it through the skin.

If Short Needle:

A 90° angle for the 5/16 inch (short) or the BD Ultra-Fine Nano needle (these hurt less and are not as likely to go into muscle)(a 90° angle looks like this: ↓)

If Longer Needle:

Use a 45° angle for the 5/8 inch needle (only)(a 45° angle looks like this: ↘)

- Push in the insulin slowly and steadily; wait 10 seconds to let the insulin spread out.

- Let go of the skin pulled up.

- Put a finger or dry cotton over the needle as it is pulled out; gently rub a few times to close the hole where the needle was inserted; press your finger or the cotton down on the area where you gave the shot if bruising or bleeding happens.

- Look to see if a drop of insulin comes back through the hole the needle made ("leak-back"); make a note in your log book if this happens.

The nurse will teach the right way to give shots so that a drop of insulin does not leak-back. A drop can contain as much as five units of insulin.

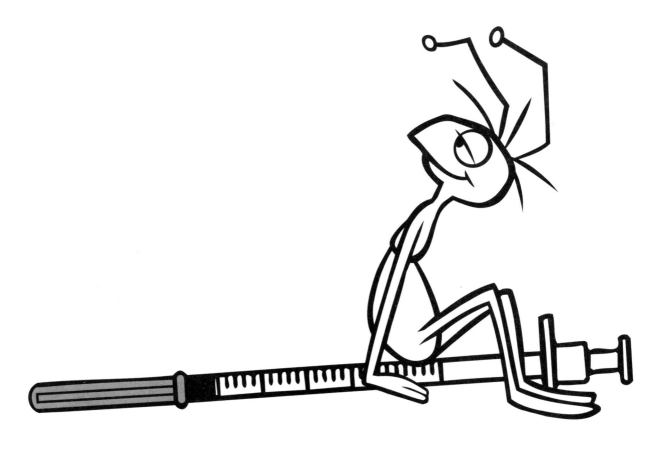

Figure 1
Drawing and Injecting the Insulin

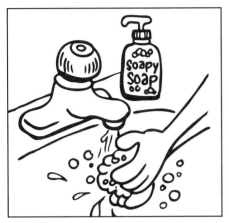

A. Wash hands

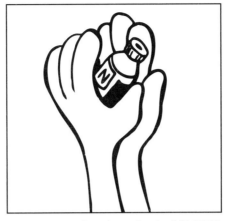

B. Warm in hands and mix (if NPH) insulin

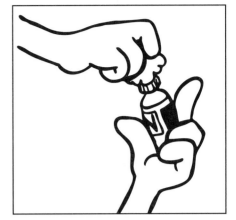

C. Wipe top of insulin bottle with alcohol

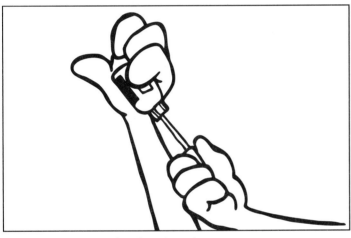

D. Inject air = insulin dose in units

Pull out dose of insulin

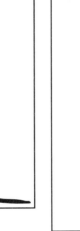

E. Make sure injection site is clean

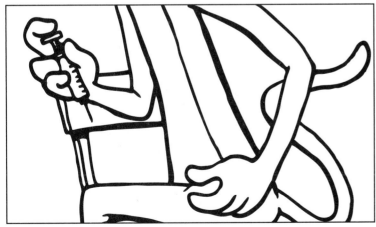

F. Pinch up skin and fat tissue. If using 5/8 inch needle, go in at angle. If using the 5/16 inch (short) or the BD Ultra-Fine Nano needle, can go straight in (assuming adequate subcutaneous fat).

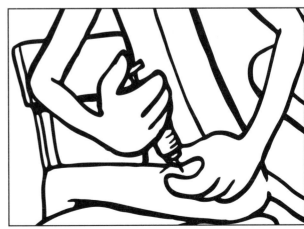

G. Basal insulins (Lantus [Basaglar], Levemir, Tresiba) are best given in the buttocks

INSULIN PENS

Insulin pens provide convenience and accuracy. Most types of insulin are now available in pens. Using a pen is quite easy and is summarized below.

- Remove the paper tab from the needle and screw it on the end of the pen.

- Clean the skin where the shot will be given. Rotate sites daily.

- Remove the needle cover.

- Enter 2 to 3 units (by rotating the dial) in the pen as a "priming dose" and with the needle pointed upward into the air, push in plunger and observe that the insulin comes out.

- Dial in the number of units to be given.

- Insert the needle under the skin.

- Inject the insulin slowly. Then count 3 seconds before removing the needle. (This prevents insulin from leaking out.)

- Rub the injection site gently to close the track of the needle.

- Put the cover back on the needle. Some say to change the needle with each injection and others say once daily.

DIFFERENT AGE CHILDREN AND INSULIN SHOTS

- A young child can help with choosing where the shot will be given (although sites must be rotated) and by holding still.

- Children usually begin to give some of their own shots around age 10.

- It is important that both mom and dad share in giving shots.

- Some age-related issues (see Chapter 18) are summarized below.

Toddlers

- This age group can sometimes be frightened when having to get shots.

- Keep the area where the shot will be given as still as possible. Try to get the child's attention on something else (e.g., television, blowing bubbles, looking at a book, etc.). This will help the child to relax.

- The buttocks are often used first, and later the legs and arms and tummy.

- With the child's permission, the Lantus [Basaglar], Levemir, Tresiba insulin can be given when the child is asleep.

- The parent must remember when giving their child a shot, they are giving them health.

School age

- The child may help in choosing the area on their body to give the shot.

- Change where the shots are given. Use two or more areas (e.g., abdomen and bottom) and use different sites within the areas (see Figure 2).

Teens

- Many teens give their own shots and do not want help.

- It is still important to give the shots in a place (e.g., the kitchen) where parents can actually see the shot given.

- Missing shots (boluses) is a common reason for poor blood sugar control.

- Parents can stay involved by helping to get the supplies out, and helping to keep records by writing down the blood sugars and insulin doses each day in the log book or by emailing meter or CGM downloads.

Figure 2

Commonly used injection sites are numbered. Rotating between sites is important to prevent swelling (hypertrophy) and altered insulin absorption.

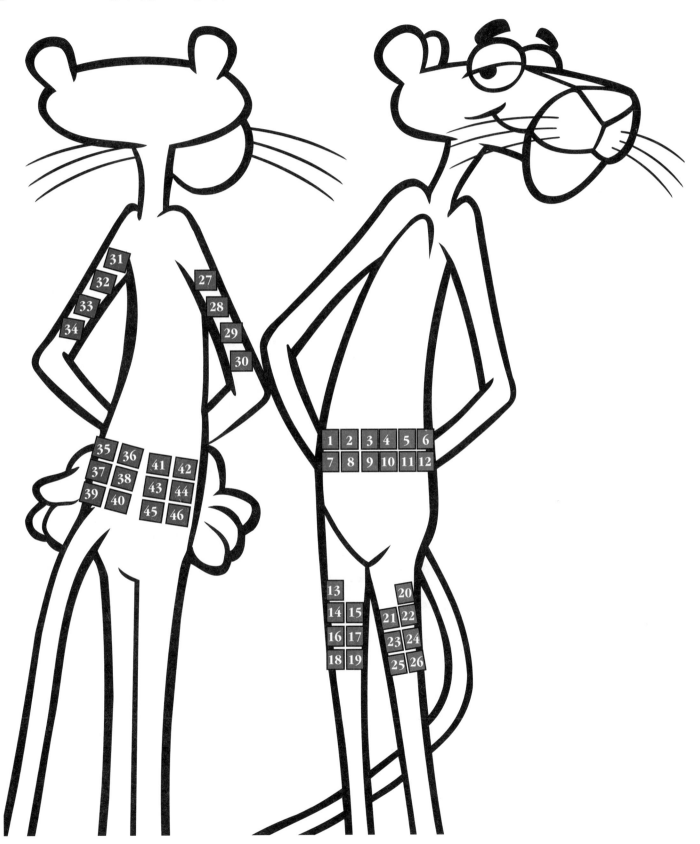

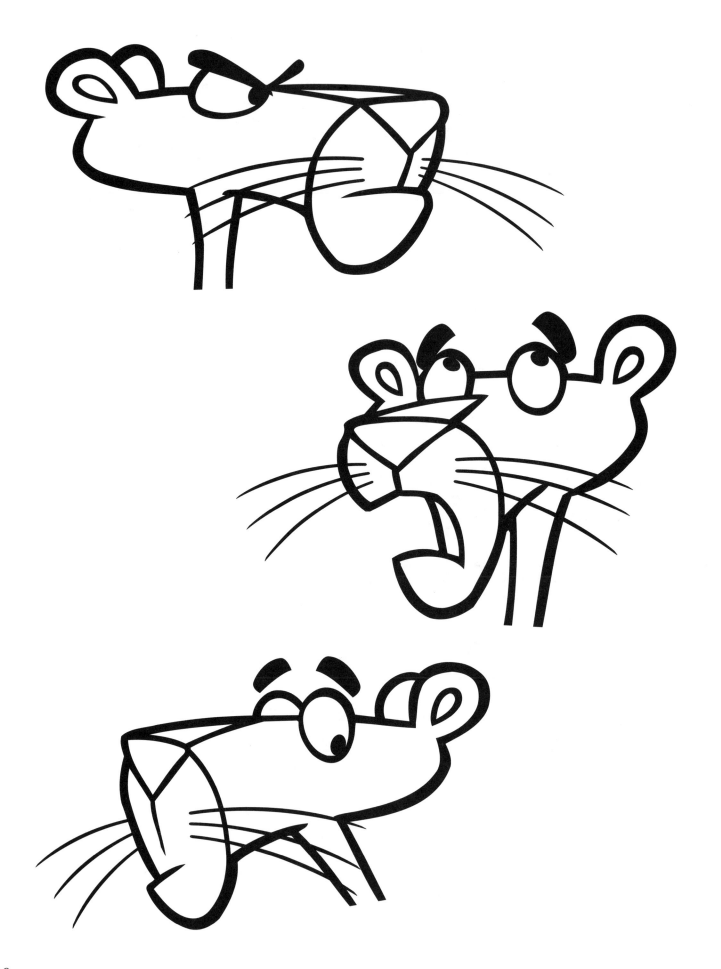

Chapter 10
Feelings/Adjustment at Diabetes Onset

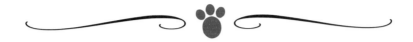

INITIAL FEELINGS

You and your child will have many feelings when you find out about diabetes. Having these feelings is very normal. It is important for families to share and talk about these feelings.

Some of the most common feelings are:

- **Shock**

- **Grief**

- **Denial**

- **Sadness**

- **Anger**

- **Fear/anxiety**

- **Guilt**

- **Adapting (as time passes, everyone will not feel so overwhelmed)**

These emotions are normal during the initial diagnosis period. Each of these feelings is discussed in detail in the larger book, *"Understanding Diabetes"* (order form in back).

We ask **EVERY** newly diagnosed family to meet with a behavioral counselor to discuss feelings. The person may be a social worker, licensed professional counselor, psychologist (a PhD), or a psychiatrist (an MD). It is important for all family members to share how they feel. All family members need to work together to learn how to fit diabetes into their lives.

As time passes, the family will find they are better able to deal with the shots, blood sugar checks, food plan and other daily tasks. Parents need to learn to share responsibilities.

ADJUSTMENT

Making life with diabetes as normal as possible is the major long-term goal. Living with diabetes will gradually become easier. Adjustment continues to improve after the first few weeks and the first few months. As time passes, the tasks below will become easier:

- Exercising daily

- Selecting healthy food choices

- Adjusting insulin for exercise

- Remembering to take insulin and/or other medications

- Checking blood sugar levels

- Counting carbohydrates

- Doing other daily diabetes-related tasks

Talking about diabetes at home and/or with the diabetes care team may help to reduce stress and create a comfortable schedule. Fitting the diabetes into as normal a lifestyle as possible becomes the major goal.

The period around initial diagnosis can be filled with many different feelings. These are normal, and tend to improve over time. Some families have recurrence of these feelings at specific times in their child's life. This will be discussed in Chapter 17.

Figure 1
What Does Your Plate for a Day Look Like?

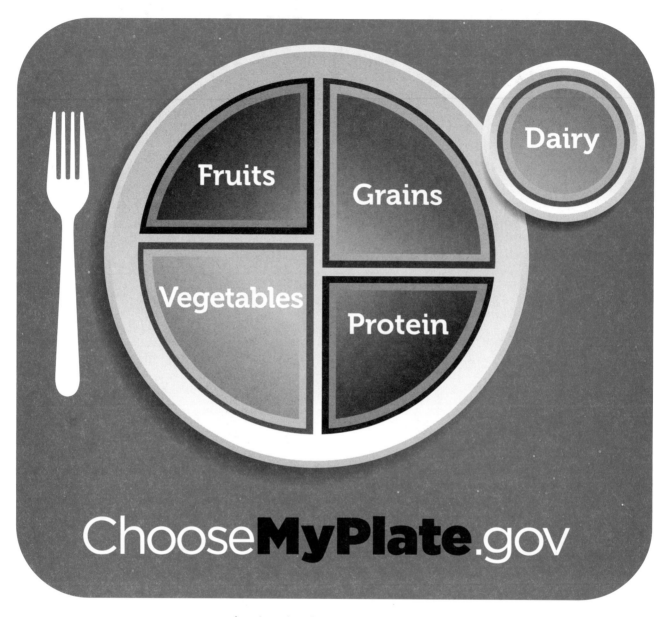

ChooseMyPlate.gov

(a helpful website)

Look at the food plate guide to see if you need to:

- eat more whole-grain foods (e.g., whole wheat bread, brown rice, cereals)

- eat more fruits and vegetables

- eat less protein and fat (particularly red meat)

Chapter 11
Normal Nutrition

Some knowledge of normal nutrition helps when working with the dietitian on a diabetes food plan. Energy from food is measured in calories.

TYPES OF FOODS

The foods we eat are divided into:

- **Proteins** – 4 calories per gram eaten

- **Carbohydrates** (includes all sugars) – 4 calories per gram eaten

- **Fats** – 9 calories per gram eaten

- **Vitamins and minerals**

- **Water**

- **Fiber**

All of these are important for our bodies and are discussed in more detail in *"Understanding Diabetes."* We emphasize with patients and families that the ideal diet for someone with diabetes is really just a healthy diet from which all people would benefit.

WEIGHT MANAGEMENT

Some people with type 2 diabetes can be treated with diet and exercise alone. This is not true for type 1 diabetes. In recent years, people with type 1 diabetes have also tended to be heavier. This results in more insulin resistance and a higher risk for heart disease. This is why snacks are no longer routinely recommended (unless on NPH insulin). **Reduction of high fat foods** and **portion control** (along with **exercise**) are important for everyone.

Foods higher in fat include:

- Red meats

- The skin of chicken or turkey

- Whole milk

- Fats and oils

- Processed foods

- Fast foods

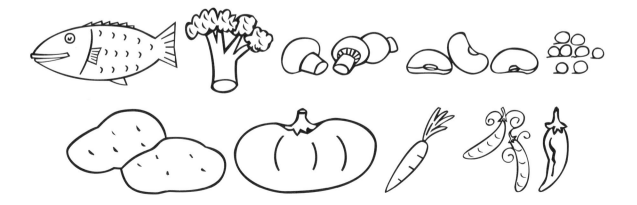

INSULIN AND CARBOHYDRATES (CARBS)

Insulin has its main effect on sugars, and a goal of treatment is matching insulin to carbohydrate intake. **It is important to think about the following:**

- **WHEN** carbohydrate is eaten.

  Snacks between meals makes blood sugar control more challenging.

- **HOW MUCH** carbohydrate is eaten. A can of sugar pop has 10 teaspoons of sugar and is unhealthy for anyone.

- **WITH WHAT** the carbohydrate is eaten. Other foods, such as fat, slow the sugar absorption.

- **IF INSULIN IS ACTING** at the same time the sugar is eaten. This allows the sugar to pass into cells for energy rather than out into the urine (see Chapter 2).

THE "PLATE" METHOD OF CHOOSING FOOD (see Figure at the beginning of this chapter)

A U.S. Department of Agriculture Center has provided an easy-to-understand guide for foods to eat. They suggest that each quarter of your plate has one of the following food groups:

- Lean protein
- Fruits
- Vegetables
- Whole-grain carbohydrate foods

Low-fat dairy products can be added.

OTHER THOUGHTS discussed in Chapter 11 of *"Understanding Diabetes"* are noted below:

- Working with the dietitian helps families keep up-to-date on new dietary ideas.

- A three-day diet record is sometimes helpful.

- Learning to read nutrition labels on foods at the store is very important.

- Having normal levels of blood fats (e.g., total cholesterol and LDL cholesterol) is important for all people. These levels can be checked every three to five years at a clinic visit; they should be checked at least yearly if they are abnormal. See Table in Chapter 23 for desired levels.

- Sugar-containing drinks such as soda are a source of "empty calories" and are unhealthy for all. They contribute to obesity and cause high blood sugar levels in people with diabetes.

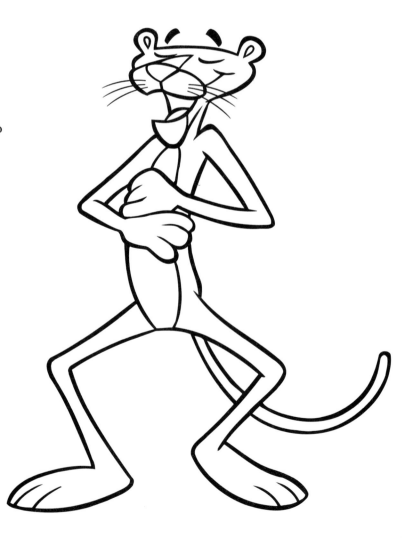

Eating nutritious foods will help all family members.

Chapter 12
Food Management and Diabetes

A food plan is important for people with either type 1 or type 2 diabetes. Every family must work out a plan with their dietitian that fits their family. As shown in the diagram in Chapter 14, food and exercise are two of the four major influences on sugar control. Both are important if excess weight is present or is to be avoided. Daily monitoring of the effects of foods on sugar levels can be done with regular blood sugar checking (see Chapter 7) or with use of a continuous glucose monitor (CGM; see Chapter 29).

People with type 1 diabetes <u>cannot</u> be treated with diet alone.

People with type 2 diabetes can sometimes be treated with diet and exercise alone. They generally need to eat foods with fewer calories and choose smaller portion sizes to reach optimal weight.

All people with diabetes should focus on a healthy, balanced diet (see Chapter 12 in *"Understanding Diabetes"*) and need to:

- Avoid sugary liquids (such as sugar pop and juices) and foods with added sugars.

- Limit meals high in added sugar, especially in the morning.

- Avoid unhealthy choices at fast food restaurants (burger, fries, pizza).

- Eat more fruits and vegetables (half of plate).

- Eat more whole grains, such as brown rice or whole-grain bread instead of white rice or white bread.

- Exercise at least 60 minutes daily.

TYPES OF FOOD PLANS

The two types of food plans that our Clinic uses the most are outlined below. Both plans require learning how to count (or estimate) carbohydrates (which are the main food source increasing blood/CGM sugar levels).

Constant carbohydrate: A person/family often starts with this plan.

- This plan involves eating about the same amount of carbs for each meal and for each snack from day to day.

- Insulin doses are changed based on the blood/CGM sugar levels, exercise, and other factors such as illness, stress, menses, etc. ("thinking scale").

Carbohydrate ("carb") counting: We encourage families to move to this plan as soon as possible. The plan involves counting the grams of carbohydrate (carbs) in food to be eaten. An amount of rapid-acting insulin is given that matches the number of grams (g) of carbohydrate (I/C ratio = insulin to carb ratio). Other parameters relating to starting carb counting are outlined below.

- The dietitian may want a three-day diet record to be done first (see Chapter 11 in *"Understanding Diabetes"*).

- The healthcare team and family initially determine the insulin-to-carb ratio (I/C ratio) for each time of day.

- The ratio used when starting this plan depends on the patient. A common starting example is one unit of insulin for each 15g of carbohydrate (I/C ratio of 1 to 15).

Table 1
How to Adjust I/C Ratios

Evaluate blood/CGM glucose levels 2 to 4 hours after a mealtime insulin dose when no correction dose was needed.

For our example: Starting I/C ratio is 1 to 15.

- If the blood/CGM sugar level is high two hours after eating (e.g., over 180 mg/dL or 10.0 mmol/L), the ratio could be changed to give more insulin for meals. In our example, change to one unit of insulin for 10g of carbs (I/C ratio of 1 to 10).

- If the blood/CGM sugar level is low two hours after eating (e.g., less than 60 mg/dL or 3.3 mmol/L), the ratio could be changed to give less insulin for meals. In our example, change to one unit of insulin for 20g of carbs (I/C ratio of 1 to 20).

- Blood/CGM glucose levels are then evaluated 2 to 4 hours after meals to see if the I/C ratio is correct (see Table 1 for example).

- Gradually, the correct ratios for each meal are found. The I/C ratio may vary for each meal.

- The blood/CGM sugar level is monitored and an insulin dose "correction factor" (see Chapter 22) is used to adjust the dose. The insulin for food (I/C ratio) plus the correction dose will be the total dose of insulin to be given 20 minutes before the meal or snack.

- If blood/CGM sugar levels are above the desired upper level one or two hours after meals (and the pre-meal blood sugar level is above 80 mg/dL [4.5 mmol/L]), it may be helpful to give the pre-meal rapid-acting insulin 20 minutes before meals. This is because sugar levels peak 60 minutes after a meal, whereas Humalog/NovoLog/Apidra insulin activity does not peak until 90 minutes after injection.

Several tables of the carb contents of foods and more details about carb counting are found in Chapter 12 of the book *"Understanding Diabetes."*

BEDTIME SNACKS

People often ask if bedtime snacks are needed. If a person has had heavy exercise, or if the blood/CGM sugar level is below 130 mg/dL (7.2 mmol/L), or if a peaking insulin (e.g., NPH) is taken at night, then make sure a bedtime snack that has solid protein, fat and carbohydrate is eaten. Otherwise, if a basal insulin is used, and the blood/CGM sugar level is above 130 mg/dL (>7.2 mmol/L) and there has not been heavy exercise, a bedtime snack may not be required as it can lead to unhealthy weight gain.

HELPFUL SUGGESTIONS FOR FOOD MANAGEMENT

Some beginning suggestions for food management, some of which relate more to a constant carb food plan, are:

- Avoid concentrated sweets
- Limit meals high in added sugar, especially in the morning
- Eat well-balanced meals
- Eat meals and snacks at approximately the same time each day
- Watch the portion size of foods to be eaten
- Snacks may be needed to prevent low blood sugars, especially with exercise (see suggested snacks in Chapter 12 of "Understanding Diabetes"). Reducing insulin as needed for exercise rather than eating extra snacks will be better for weight control.
- Avoid over-treating low blood sugars (see Chapter 6)
- Eat foods with less cholesterol, saturated fats and trans-fats
- Monitor for appropriate growth
- Watch weight for height; avoid becoming overweight
- Increase the amount of fiber eaten
- Eat fewer foods that are high in salt (sodium)
- Complete dietary guidelines are available at **www.dietaryguidelines.gov**

Table 2
Six Dietary Factors to Aid with Sugar Control*

1. Follow some sort of a meal plan
2. Avoid high-carb meals, especially in the morning
3. Avoid over-treating low blood sugars (hypoglycemia)
4. Adjust insulin levels for meals
5. Avoid eating extra snacks
6. Promptly treat high blood/CGM sugar levels when found

* From the **DCCT**: Diabetes Control and Complications Trial (see Chapter 14)

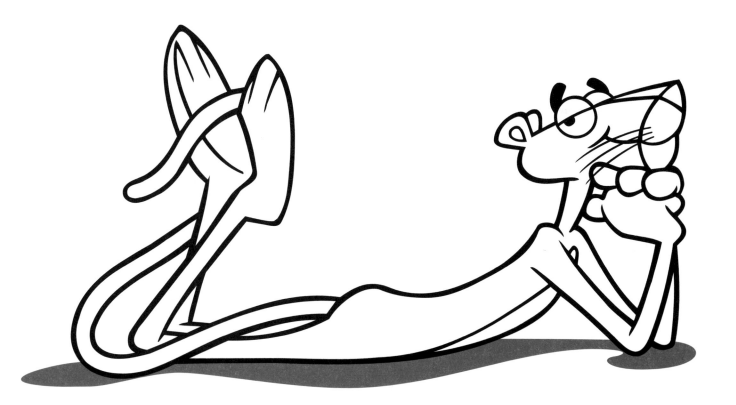

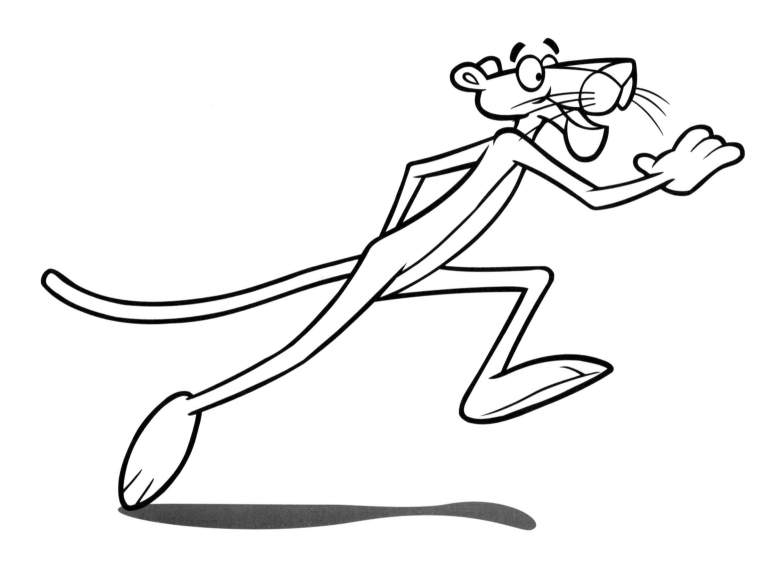

Getting plenty of exercise is important for everyone.

Chapter 13
Exercise and Diabetes

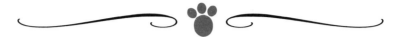

Regular exercise is important for everyone. It may be even more important for people with diabetes. For people with type 2 diabetes, regular exercise and eating less food are two of the most important parts of treating the diabetes (see Chapter 4). Many high-performing and professional athletes have diabetes (see *"Understanding Diabetes,"* Chapter 13). These athletes do not let diabetes get in the way of success and enjoying their sports.

Exercise may result in lower or higher (usually due to excess snacks) blood/CGM sugar levels. Overall, exercise helps to keep the blood/CGM sugar values in the target range. It does this in part by making the body more sensitive to insulin.

EXERCISE:

• Is one of the "big four," along with insulin (or oral medicines), food and stress, which affect blood sugar levels (see Figure 2 in Chapter 14)

Figure

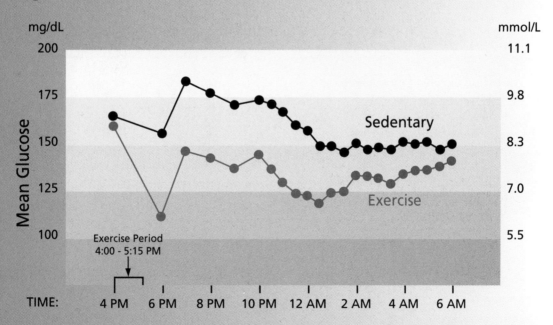

Blood Sugars With and Without One Hour of Exercise

Exercise has a prolonged impact on blood sugars. This Figure presents blood glucose (sugar) levels for the same 50 children with type 1 diabetes on a sedentary day (black circles) and an exercise day (red circles). One hour of exercise at 4 p.m. resulted in lower blood sugar levels for the next 14 hours (through the night). Insulin doses and food intake were identical for the two days.

(Data compliments of the DirecNet Study Group: J Pediatr 147, 528, 2005)

- Is essential for weight control and is a primary part of treating type 2 diabetes

- Should be done daily for 60 minutes by people with type 1 or type 2 diabetes (and by all people)

- Generally lowers blood sugar levels (see Figure)

- Requires extra fluids during exercise to prevent dehydration

PREVENTING LOWS

Exercise can cause **low blood/CGM sugar values** (Chapter 6) so it is important to plan ahead. If a low blood sugar does occur, it is important to stop the exercise, treat the low blood sugar, and not resume exercise until the blood/CGM sugar level is back up. The following may help to prevent lows:

- Extra snacks or less insulin may be needed. When possible, such as when using an insulin pump, stop or reduce insulin for heavy exercise instead of increasing snacks. This will help lead to a healthier weight.

- Aiming for a higher blood/CGM sugar level before exercise (e.g., 180 mg/dL [10.0 mmol/L])

- Rechecking extra blood/CGM sugar levels (e.g., during and after exercise)

- Use of drinks (such as Gatorade®) during vigorous exercise

- Thinking ahead to prevent low blood sugars for up to 24 hours after the exercise ("delayed hypoglycemia") by means such as:

    ◊ The evening insulin dose may need to be reduced

    ◊ Adding an extra 15 or 30 grams of carbohydrate at bedtime if afternoon or evening exercise has been strenuous (without taking extra insulin)

    ◊ Making sure the bedtime blood/CGM glucose value is above 130 mg/dL (7.2 mmol/L)

- Noticing the impact different sports have on your body and your blood sugar levels. Some people experience more lows with certain sports than with others.

INSULIN PUMPS

- Use of an insulin pump and/or CGM makes insulin adjustments easier in preventing exercise-related hypoglycemia.

- Using reduced temporary basal rates before, during and after exercise can be helpful (Chapter 28).

- Some insulin-pump users who disconnect from their pump for long periods during exercise can benefit by giving part of their basal insulin as Lantus (Basaglar) or Levemir and part via the pump. For example, half of the basal insulin could be given by the pump (50% temp basal for 24 hours) and the other half given as a shot of one of the above basal insulins. There would then be some insulin activity while disconnected from the pump.

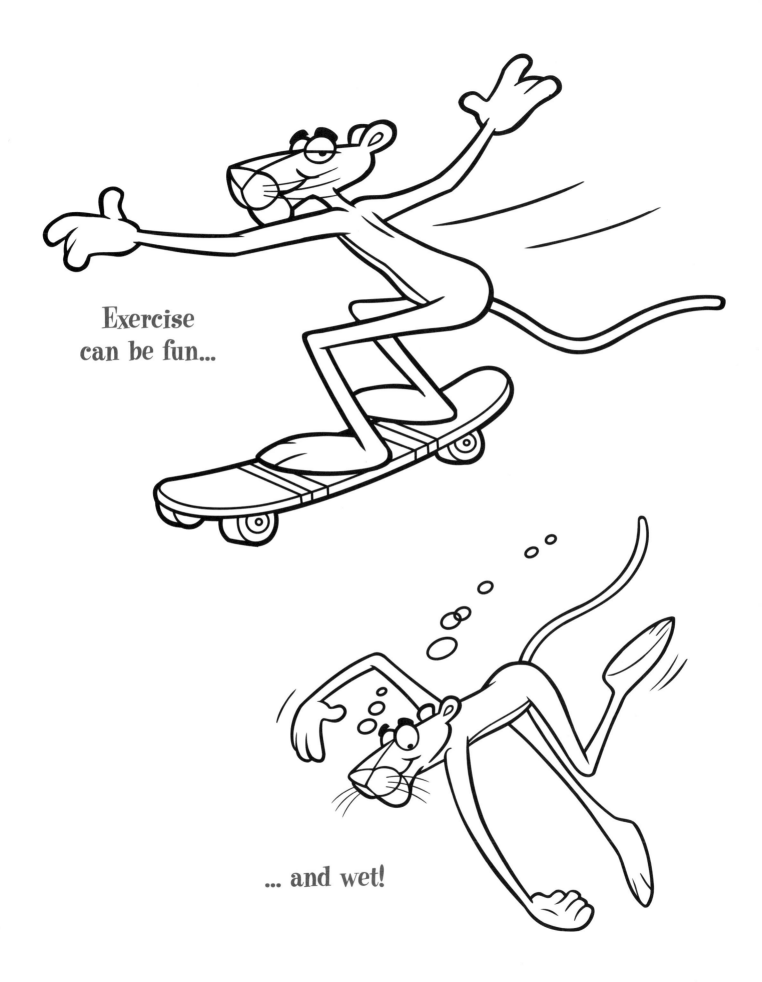

Exercise
can be fun...

... and wet!

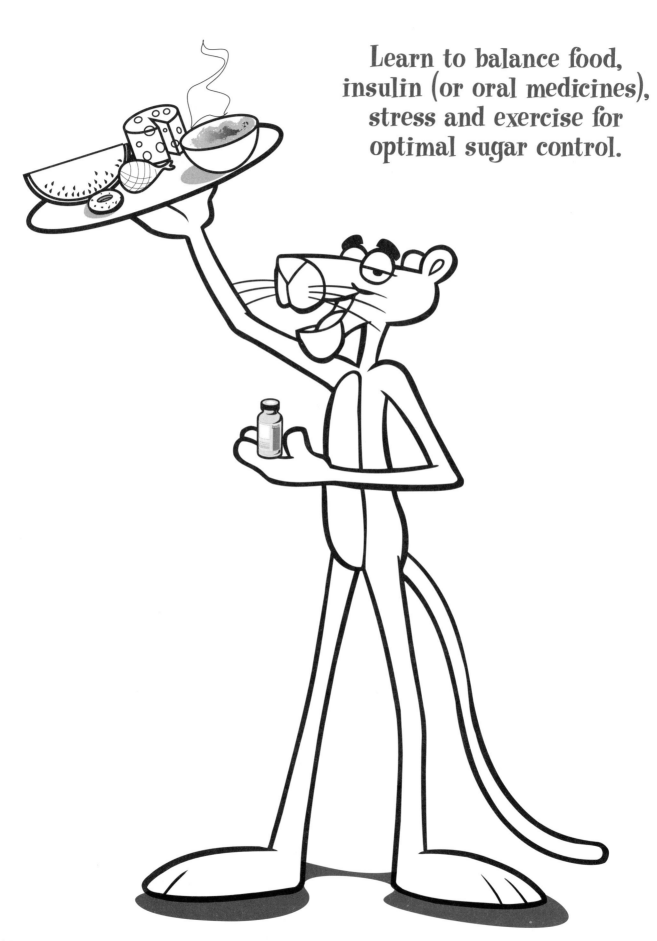

Learn to balance food, insulin (or oral medicines), stress and exercise for optimal sugar control.

Chapter 14
Monitoring Diabetes Control

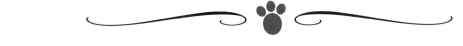

A goal for the management of diabetes is to have blood/CGM sugar levels as close to the levels of someone without diabetes as is safely possible. At least half of all values should be "in-range" for age (see Table).

SUGAR* CONTROL:

- Is measured day-to-day by checking blood sugar levels on a meter or by a continuous glucose monitor (CGM; see Chapter 29)

- Is monitored for the longer term by a very important measurement called the hemoglobin A1c (**HbA1c or A1c; see Figure 1**)

THE HbA1c (A1c) VALUE:

- Can be thought of as the **"forest"** and the blood/CGM sugar values as the **"trees"**

- Increases when blood/CGM sugars have been high (see Figure 1)

- Tells how often the sugars have been high for the past 90 days

- Should be done every three months

- Is now recommended to be below 7.5% (58 mmol/mol) for all children and adolescents

The best goal is to have an HbA1c as low as possible (no lower than 6.0% [42 mmol/mol]), balanced with infrequent hypoglycemia and a high quality of life. Having an HbA1c too low may result in excessive hypoglycemia.

BLOOD/ CGM SUGAR LEVELS**

- Ranges for blood/CGM sugar values should be set for every person (see Table).

- Meters and CGMs can usually be downloaded to a computer to provide the percent of values in-range, high and low. This data should be reviewed at least weekly. Aim for over 50 percent of values in-range (Table) and no more than 10 percent low.

- Meters and CGMs can usually display 7, 14 or 30-day averages. These can be used to know if dose changes are working or if more changes are needed. If using a CGM, knowing the average glucose level is very important in evaluating sugar control.

- Sugar control is influenced by four major factors (Figure 2).

---

* In this book, the words "sugar" and "glucose" are used to have the same meaning.

** When the term "blood/CGM" is used, it indicates the sugar may have been measured from a blood sample or by a continuous glucose monitor (CGM).

WHY IS SUGAR CONTROL IMPORTANT?

Optimal sugar control:

- Helps people feel better

- Can lessen the future risk for eye, kidney, nerve and heart problems from diabetes. This was proven by The DCCT (Diabetes Control and Complications Trial)

- Helps to lower blood fats (cholesterol and triglyceride levels; see Chapter 11)

- Includes reduction of the wide "swings" (variability) in blood/CGM sugar levels

- Helps children grow to their full adult height

- Reduces the risks for diabetic ketoacidosis (DKA; Chapter 15) and severe hypoglycemia (see Chapter 6)

- Is a reflection of the balancing of food, insulin (or oral meds), exercise and stress (see Figure 2)

A lower HbA1c is better (<7.5% or 58 mmol/mol), but this must be balanced with a good quality of life and infrequent hypoglycemia.

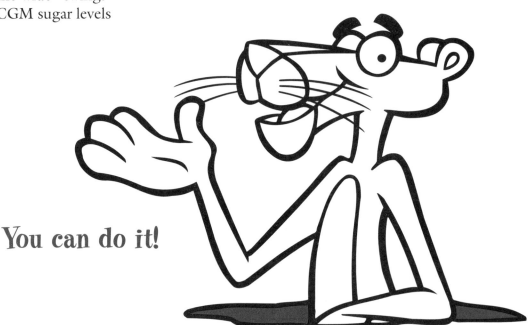

You can do it!

Table

Desired Ranges for Someone with Diabetes			
	Hemoglobin A1c	Blood/CGM Glucose: mg/dL (mmol/L)*	
	HbA1c: % (mmol/mol)*	Fasting/ Before Meals*	Bedtime/Overnight
0-5 years	<7.5% (<58)	70-150 (3.9-8.3)	100-180 (5.5-10.0)
6-17 years	<7.5% (<58)	70-130 (3.9-7.2)	90-150 (5.0-8.3)
18 years and up	<7.0% (<53)	70-130 (3.9-7.2)	90-150 (5.0-8.3)

< = less than; > =greater than

† After heavy exercise, a goal of 130-150 (7.2-8.3) might be a safer level at bedtime.

* Values in parentheses represent mmol/L (glucose) or mmol/mol (HbA1c). The HbA1c levels are as recommended by the ADA in 2014.

Figure 1

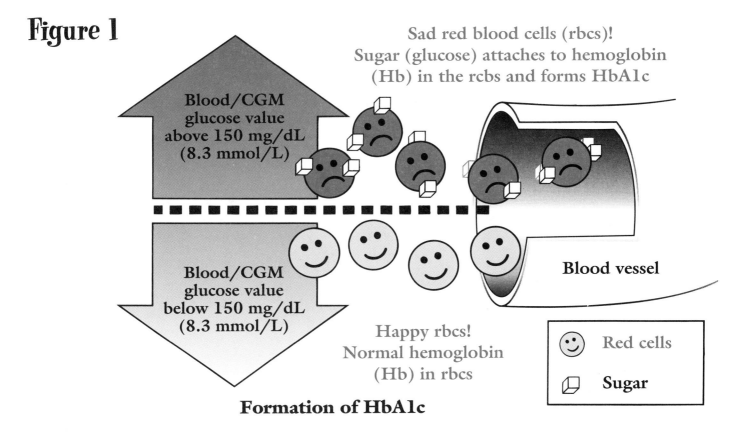

Sad red blood cells (rbcs)!
Sugar (glucose) attaches to hemoglobin
(Hb) in the rcbs and forms HbA1c

Blood/CGM
glucose value
above 150 mg/dL
(8.3 mmol/L)

Blood/CGM
glucose value
below 150 mg/dL
(8.3 mmol/L)

Blood vessel

Happy rbcs!
Normal hemoglobin
(Hb) in rbcs

😊	Red cells
▱	**Sugar**

Formation of HbA1c

Figure 2

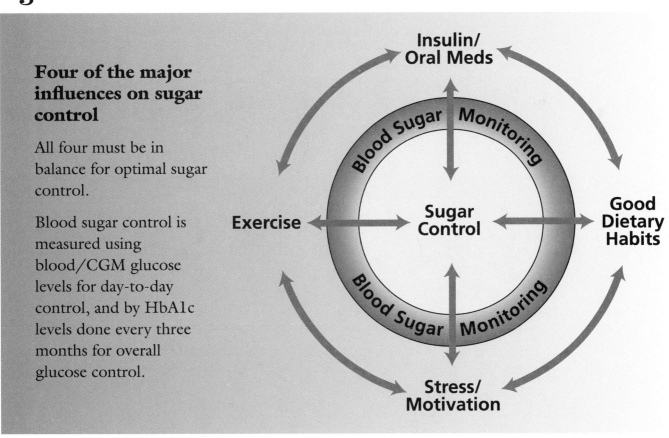

Four of the major influences on sugar control

All four must be in balance for optimal sugar control.

Blood sugar control is measured using blood/CGM glucose levels for day-to-day control, and by HbA1c levels done every three months for overall glucose control.

Insulin/
Oral Meds

Blood Sugar Monitoring

Exercise

Sugar
Control

Good
Dietary
Habits

Blood Sugar Monitoring

Stress/
Motivation

Table

Comparison of the Two Emergencies of Diabetes

	Low Blood Sugar (Chapter 6) (Hypoglycemia or Insulin Reaction)	Ketoacidosis (Chapter 15) (Acidosis or DKA)
Due to:	Low blood sugar	Presence of ketones
Time of onset:	Fast – within minutes	Slow – in hours or days
Causes:	Too little food Too much insulin Too much exercise without food Missing or being late for meals/snacks Excitement in young children	Too little insulin Not giving insulin Infections/Illness Traumatic body stress Pump insertions malfunctioning
Blood sugar:	Low (below 70 mg/dL or 3.9 mmol/L)	Usually high (over 240 mg/dL or 13.3 mmol/L)
Ketones:	Usually none in the urine or blood	Usually moderate/large in the urine or blood ketones over 0.6 mmol/L.

	SYMPTOMS	TREATMENT	SYMPTOMS	TREATMENT
Mild:	Hunger, shaky, sweaty, nervous	Give juice or milk. Wait 15 minutes and recheck B.S. Repeat as needed	Thirst, frequent urination, sweet breath, small or moderate urine ketones or blood ketones less than 1.0 mmol/L.	Give lots of fluids and Humalog/NovoLog/Apidra or Regular insulin every two or three hours.
Moderate:	Headache, unexpected behavior changes, impaired or double vision, confusion, drowsiness, weakness or difficulty talking.	Give Insta-Glucose or a fast-acting sugar, juice or sugar pop (4 oz). After 15 minutes, recheck B.S. Repeat as needed	Dry mouth, nausea, stomach cramps, vomiting, moderate or large urine ketones or blood ketones between 1.0 and 3.0 mmol/L.	Continued contact with healthcare-provider. Give lots of fluids. Give Humalog/NovoLog/Apidra or Regular insulin every two or three hours. Give Zofran (a tablet) or Phenergan medication (suppository or topical cream) if vomiting occurs. *
Severe:	Loss of consciousness or seizures occurs after being low for a prolonged time.	Give glucagon (by shot or inhaled). Check blood sugar. If no response, call paramedic (911) or go to E.R.	Labored deep breathing, extreme weakness, confusion and eventually unconsciousness (coma), large urine ketones or blood ketones above 3.0 mmol/L.	*Go to the emergency room.* May need intravenous fluids and insulin.

*Note: If these medications are given, a helper must assist to make sure blood sugar and ketones are checked frequently, as the patient will be sleepy.

Chapter 15
Ketones and Diabetic Ketoacidosis (DKA)

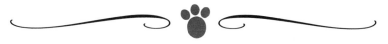

This is the second emergency for people with diabetes (the other being low blood sugar, Chapter 6). DKA is more common in people with type 1 compared to type 2 diabetes, but can occur in type 2 diabetes. Low blood sugar is more common than DKA, although episodes of DKA are more dangerous. DKA is generally easy to differentiate from low blood sugar (see Table).

WHAT LEADS TO DKA?

DKA occurs when ketones build up in the body because there isn't enough insulin. DKA is avoidable in a person with known diabetes.

Ketones are:

* Made by the body when there is not enough insulin in the body, so sugar cannot be used for energy.

* Acids that form when the body breaks down fat for the energy it needs.

* Dangerous when present in high amounts.

HOW DOES IT START?

* The body makes ketones when there isn't enough insulin. Ketones can be measured in the urine or blood (see Chapter 5).

* The longer the body doesn't get the insulin it needs, the higher the ketone (acid) level. Excess ketones result in **DKA** (**D**iabetic **K**eto**A**cidosis).

WHAT ARE THE MAIN CAUSES OF INCREASED KETONES OR OF DKA?

* Forgetting to give one or more insulin shots is the most common cause of DKA in patients with known diabetes.

* Illness: the amount of insulin usually needs to be increased from the person's normal doses so the body will have the extra energy from carbohydrates needed to fight the illness. Otherwise, fat is broken down to provide energy, and ketones rise. This is why we recommend checking ketones with all illnesses. Sometimes during illness, ketones can develop even when blood/CGM sugar levels haven't been especially high. They are more apt to occur when there is poor appetite, vomiting or diarrhea.

* Not enough insulin (dose too small) may result in ketone build-up.

* An insulin pump that is not delivering insulin (usually due to kinked, obstructed or dislodged infusion catheter) may result in ketones in three hours. Children, ages 9 years and younger, may produce ketones when insulin has not been delivered for two or more hours.

* Giving "spoiled" insulin (insulin that got too hot [over 90° F, 32° C] or froze) can be a cause of increased ketones.

* Traumatic stress on the body (particularly for people with type 2 diabetes) may cause ketones.

DKA can be very dangerous. It usually does not occur unless large urine ketones or high blood ketones (above 3.0 mmol/L) have been present for several hours. See the Table for advice on treatment of different levels of ketones. It can be avoided in people with known diabetes by checking blood or urine ketones as instructed (see following).

WHAT ARE THE SIGNS OF DKA?

- Thirst and frequent urination are common due to the associated high blood/CGM sugar levels.

- A stomachache, vomiting, or a sweet or fruity odor to the breath (like acetone, or nail polish remover) can occur with high ketones.

- If large urine ketones or blood ketones above 3.0 mmol/L have been present for many hours, deep or rapid breathing can occur or a person may seem confused, less alert or hard to wake up. These are late signs of DKA. You need to go to the emergency room immediately!

WHEN SHOULD KETONES BE CHECKED?

Check for blood or urine ketones (see methods in Chapter 5):

- With any illness **(even vomiting one time)**

- Anytime two or more blood/CGM sugar levels are above 300 mg/dL (16.7 mmol/L) at any time during the day

- Anytime the first morning blood/CGM glucose level is above 300 mg/dL (16.7 mmol/L)

- With a pump infusion set failure

- When a basal insulin shot has been missed

TREATMENT OF ELEVATED KETONES

- It is important to drink extra liquids. The extra liquids help to wash out the ketones and prevent dehydration.

- When ketones are high, it is best to NOT exercise as the ketone level may increase.

- It is important to keep the blood/CGM sugar level up (e.g., above 100 mg/dL [5.5 mmol/L]) so that enough insulin can be given to turn off ketone production without having low blood sugar (see Chapter 16 on Sick Day Management).

- If help is needed, call the diabetes care-provider when moderate or large urine ketones are found, or if the blood ketones are above 1.0 mmol/L.

- Extra doses of rapid-acting insulin (by shot if using an insulin pump) will be needed every two hours until the high blood ketones or the moderate or large urine ketones are gone. The family can make repeat calls every two hours to the doctor or nurse if help is needed.

- If trouble breathing, confusion, or if excessive vomiting occurs, you need to go to the Emergency Department.

We have found that DKA can be prevented 95 percent of the time in a person with known diabetes if the instructions in this chapter are followed.

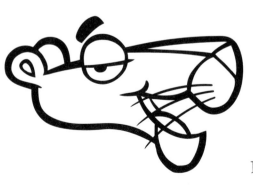

Drinking fluids helps remove ketones from the body.

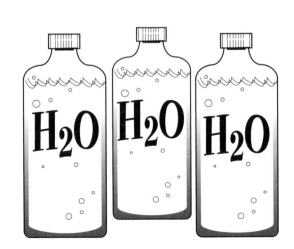

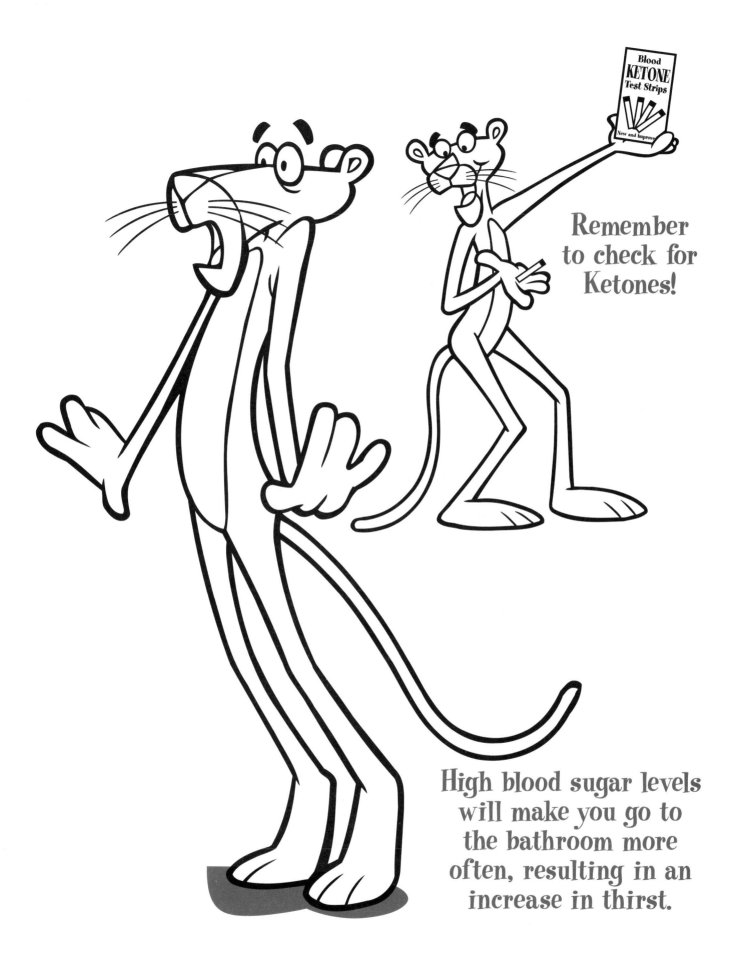

Remember
to check for
Ketones!

High blood sugar levels
will make you go to
the bathroom more
often, resulting in an
increase in thirst.

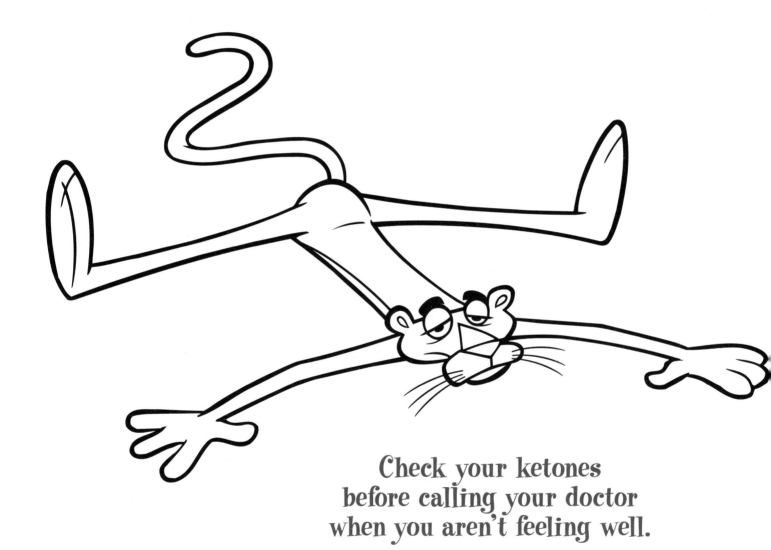

Check your ketones
before calling your doctor
when you aren't feeling well.

Chapter 16
Sick Day/Surgery Management

SICK DAY MANAGEMENT

People with diabetes get sick just like other people. For example, the average child gets six to eight colds a year. Illnesses may affect diabetes management. More frequent blood sugar checking and/or use of the continuous glucose monitor (CGM) can be very helpful during times of illness.

Ketones

- Always check **urine and/or blood ketones** (see Chapter 5) and the **blood/CGM sugar levels** with any illness. Check ketones even if the blood sugar level is normal.

- The earlier you treat the ketones with extra Humalog/NovoLog/Apidra (or Regular) insulin and fluids, the less chance you will have to go into the hospital. If using an insulin pump, repeat injections (not by pump) are given every two hours until the ketones are below moderate in the urine or below 0.6 mmol/L in the blood. We do not recommend treating elevated ketones by insulin pump, as the tubing may be plugged.

- Call your diabetes doctor or nurse if the urine ketone result is moderate or large or if the blood ketone level is above 1.0 mmol/L and you need assistance (see Chapter 15 on prevention of DKA).

Insulin

- If vomiting is present and ketones are negative, the insulin dose may have to be lowered, but **some insulin must still be given.** Ketones usually start to form after three hours without insulin, but may appear in less time when the person is sick or in children under ten years old (especially after a pump suspension of two hours or more).

- If the person vomits three or more times, some doctors will prescribe a Phenergan suppository (or skin-application) or orally dissolved tablets called Zofran®. Children under two years of age should not use a Phenergan suppository. Phenergan and Zofran may cause drowsiness. For this reason, the person will need assistance to make sure blood/CGM sugar or urine ketones are checked every 2-3 hours if these medications are used. Other information related to handling vomiting is given in Table 1.

Low-Dose Glucagon

- A low-dose may be helpful when the blood/CGM sugar level is low and vomiting continues (see Chapter 6).

- Glucagon can be mixed and given with an insulin syringe just like insulin.

- The dose of glucagon is much lower than the dose given for severe hypoglycemia.

- The dose is one unit for every year of age up to 15 units.

- It should <u>not</u> be given if urine ketones are moderate or large (or blood ketones above 1.0 mmol/L).

- The glucagon can be repeated every 20 minutes if needed.

- If available, intra-nasal glucagon can be used instead of the injection.

Table 1
Management of Vomiting (without ketones)

- Avoid solid foods until the vomiting has stopped.

- If vomiting is frequent, some doctors recommend giving a Phenergan suppository (or skin application) or an orally dissolved tablet called Zofran to reduce vomiting. It may be best to wait for an hour until the medicine is working before giving fluids. Children under two years of age should not use a Phenergan suppository. If you use these medications, the blood/CGM sugar and ketone monitoring directions must be followed (see text).

- Gradually start liquids (juice, Pedialyte®, water, etc.) in small amounts. Juices (especially orange) replace the salts that are lost with vomiting or diarrhea. Pedialyte popsicles are also available.

- Start with a tablespoon of liquid every 10-20 minutes.

- If the blood/CGM glucose level is below 100 mg/dL (5.5 mmol/L) sugar pop or other liquids containing sugar can be given.

- If the blood /CGM sugar level is below 70 mg/dL (3.9 mmol/L) and the person is vomiting, give a low-dose injection of glucagon just as you would give insulin. The dose is 1 unit per year of age up to 15 units (see text). Repeat doses can be given every 20 minutes as needed. If available, intra-nasal glucagon can be used instead of injectable glucagon.

- If the blood/CGM sugar level is above 150 mg/dL (8.3 mmol/L), do not give pop or other drinks with sugar.

- If there is no further vomiting, gradually increase the amount of fluid.

- If vomiting restarts, it may again be necessary to rest the stomach for another hour and then restart the small amounts of fluids. A repeat Phenergan suppository or Zofran tablet can be given after three or four hours.

- After a few hours without vomiting, gradually return to a normal diet. Soups are often helpful to start with and they provide needed nutrients.

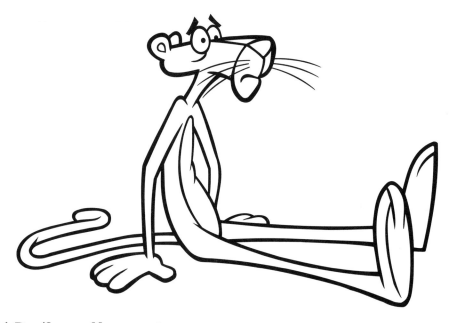

Other Medications/Foods/Care

Many medications have a warning label that a person with diabetes should not use the medicine. This is often because they may raise the blood/CGM glucose levels a few points.

- If this is the case, go ahead and take it. The insulin dose can be adjusted.

- Steroids (e.g., prednisone) may cause very high blood/CGM sugar levels and are often used for asthma or croup. If prescribed, the diabetes care-provider should be notified.

- Suggestions for sick day foods are given in Table 2.

- People with diabetes who have complications (eye, kidney, nerve, or heart disease) may need to avoid some medications.

- Table 3 may help you decide when and whom to call for extra help.

Type 2 Diabetes

Youth with type 2 diabetes must also remember to check the urine and/or blood ketone level with any illness.

- If the person is receiving metformin (Glucophage), the pills should be stopped during the illness.

- It may be best to return to insulin shots during the illness.

- Call your doctor or nurse if you have questions.

SURGERY MANAGEMENT

If surgery is planned, call your diabetes care-provider AFTER you find out the time of the surgery and whether eating food in usual amounts will be allowed.

Take your own diabetes supplies with you to the surgery, including:

- Blood sugar meter and strips, with finger poker (lancet)

- CGM (if used) and extra sensor

- Insulin and syringes

- Glucose (dextrose) tablets or gel

- Blood ketone strips and meter or urine Ketostix

- Glucagon emergency kit or (if available) intra-nasal glucagon

- If on a pump, equipment to change infusion set if needed and extra insulin

- Your phone card with your diabetes care-provider's number

If you receive a basal insulin (e.g., by insulin pump or by Lantus [Basaglar], Levemir or Tresiba injection), the basal insulin can be continued during the period of surgery. Some people who tend to have low blood/CGM sugar levels can reduce the basal insulin dose by 10 to 20 percent. This should be discussed with your diabetes care-provider. Boluses by insulin pump or injections may be restarted when the person is able to eat. Be sure to speak to the surgery team about blood sugar and insulin management.

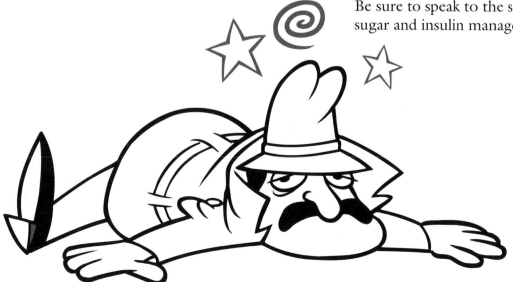

Table 2
Sick Day Foods

Liquids*

- Fruit juice: apple, cranberry, grape, grapefruit, orange, pineapple, etc.
- Sugar-containing beverages: regular 7Up®, ginger ale, orange juice, cola, PEPSI®, etc.*
- Fruit-flavored drinks: regular Kool-Aid, lemonade, Hi-C®, etc.*
- Sports drinks: Gatorade, POWERADE®, etc., any flavor
- Pedialyte, or Infalyte® (especially for younger children)
- JELL-O®: regular or diet
- Popsicles, regular or diet
- Broth-type soup: bouillon, chicken noodle soup, Cup-a-Soup®

Solids (when ready)

- Saltine crackers
- Banana (or other fruit)
- Applesauce
- Bread or toast
- Graham crackers
- Soup

* Sugar-free may be needed depending on blood/CGM glucose levels (e.g., greater than 150 mg/dL [8.3 mmol/L]).

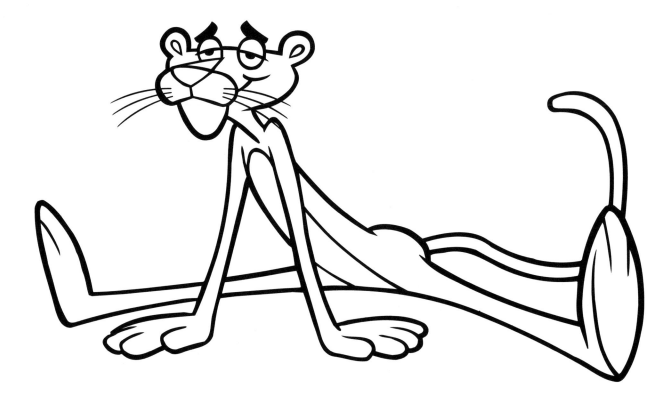

Table 3
Sick Day Management
When/Whom to Call for Emergency Care

- Call your family doctor if you have vomited three or more times and can keep nothing in your stomach, but urine ketones are not moderate or large or blood ketones above 1.0 mmol/L.

- If moderate or large ketones are present or blood ketones are above 1.0 mmol/L, call your diabetes care-provider if you have questions about treatment.

- *If help is needed with an insulin dose, call your diabetes care-provider.*

- If you have difficulty breathing or have rapid or deep breathing, you need to go to an emergency room immediately. This usually indicates severe acidosis (ketoacidosis; Chapter 15).

- Low blood sugar (hypoglycemia) can occur with vomiting or not eating normal amounts of food. More frequent blood/CGM sugar checks are important. If there is any unusual behavior such as confusion, slurred speech, double vision, inability to move or talk, or jerking, someone should give sugar or Insta-Glucose. Check the blood/CGM sugar level when possible. A shot of glucagon (Chapter 6) should be given if the person is unconscious or if a convulsion (seizure) occurs. Intra-nasal glucagon can be used instead of the injection. In case of a convulsion (seizure) or loss of consciousness, it may be necessary to call the paramedics or to go to an emergency room. Have an emergency number posted by the phone. The diabetes care-provider should be contacted if a severe reaction has occurred.

Your insulin dose may change when you are sick, but you always need some insulin.

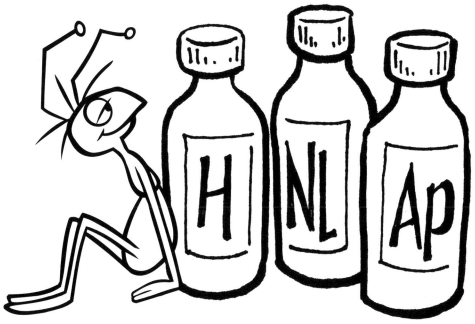

Family support
is very important
for the person
with diabetes.

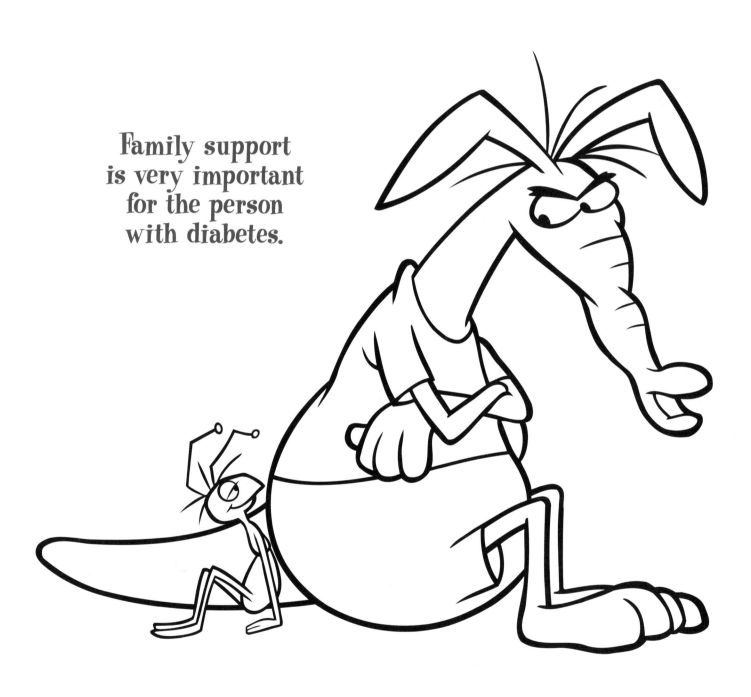

Chapter 17
Family Concerns

Diabetes is a family disease. All family members need to work together to incorporate diabetes into their lives. This means that all family members must help. The people who do best with their diabetes have the help and support of all family members.

- It is important for children with diabetes to be treated just like other children. This includes having normal boundaries, chores and consequences. A rule to follow is:

THINK OF THE CHILD FIRST AND THE DIABETES SECOND.

- It is important that all family members share their feelings (see Chapter 10).

- Siblings often feel left out when the child with diabetes needs more attention. This should be discussed with the other children, and time should be set aside for them as well.

- Perhaps the most supportive and loving act that parents, brothers and sisters can make for the person with diabetes is to remove high-sugar foods (candy, sugar soda pop, donuts, cookies, etc.) from the home. These foods have little nutritional value and are not healthy for any family members.

SPECIFIC AREAS OF CONCERN

- The stress of the diagnosis of diabetes is real for all family members. Any of the feelings discussed in Chapter 10 (e.g., sadness, anger, guilt) may linger. They generally improve with time.

- One of the four big influences on blood/CGM sugar levels is stress (see Chapter 14). The psych-social team (social worker or psychologist) is available to help in dealing with stress and other feelings.

- Extra activity and excitement may cause low (or high) blood/CGM sugar levels in people with diabetes. Some of the following may include delayed meals as well as increased activity:

  - Family picnics
  - Sleepovers
  - Trips to the beach or hiking
  - School field days or trips
  - A trip to Disney® or other theme parks
  - Special days such as Christmas, Hanukkah or Ramadan

Thinking ahead, adjusting the insulin dose, checking more blood/CGM glucose levels and giving extra snacks if sugar levels are low may result in a better day for everyone.

- Wearing a medical alert ID bracelet (or other ID) is important.

- Needle fears occur in about one-fourth of all people. The psych-social team may be helpful, particularly in suggesting distractions (TV, toys, books) or relaxation techniques (also see

Chapter 9). If family members have needle fears, the psych-social team may need to help.

- Missed shots (or insulin boluses for the pumper) result in an elevated HbA1c level and an increased risk for diabetic complications. Help from other family members, teachers, friends or counselors to remember injections may be needed.

- Driving a car when there is a risk of hypoglycemia can be a family concern relating to a person with diabetes and is discussed in Chapter 20.

- Fear of hypoglycemia is common and must be dealt with, or it may prevent optimal management of diabetes. Education or counseling may help alleviate this fear. The use of CGM (Chapter 29) is often helpful. A pump and CGM system has been approved that stops insulin infusion when a person is hypoglycemic (see Chapter 30 for more details). The artificial pancreas (Chapter 30) was also approved and has protective features to prevent hypoglycemia.

- Other behavioral issues (e.g., eating disorders) are discussed in the book, *"Understanding Diabetes."*

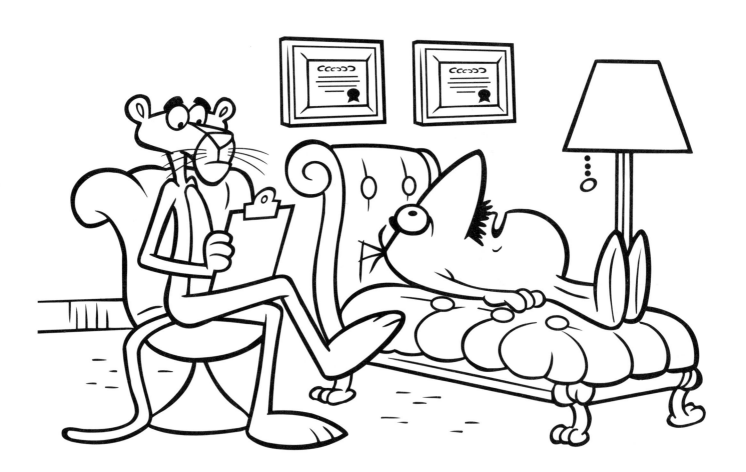

Social workers and psychologists are there to help you.

Think of the
person first and
THEN the diabetes.

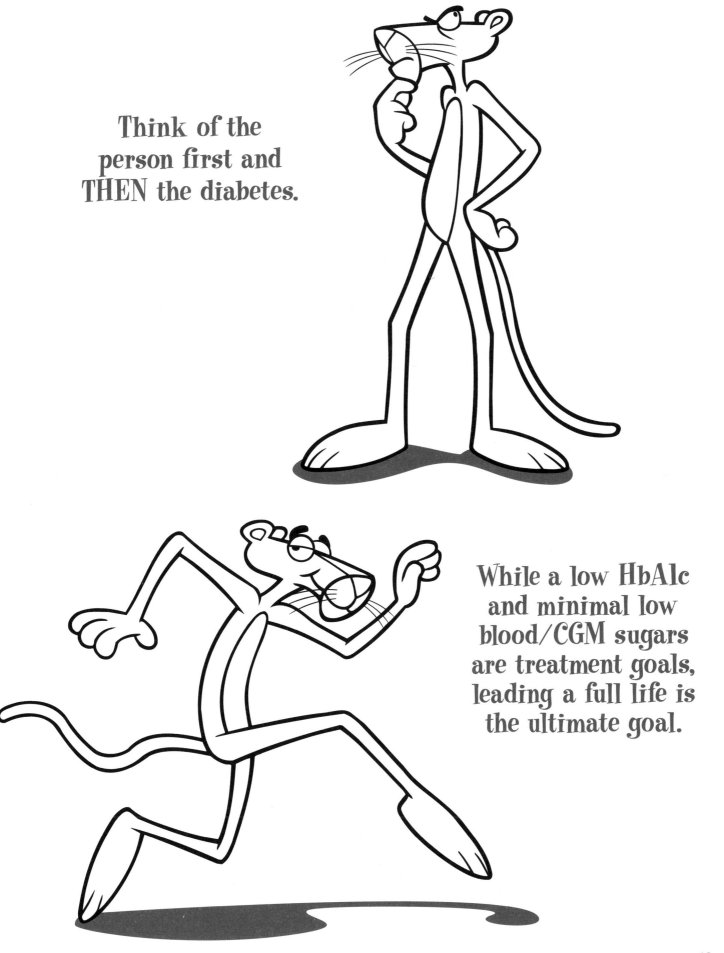

While a low HbAlc
and minimal low
blood/CGM sugars
are treatment goals,
leading a full life is
the ultimate goal.

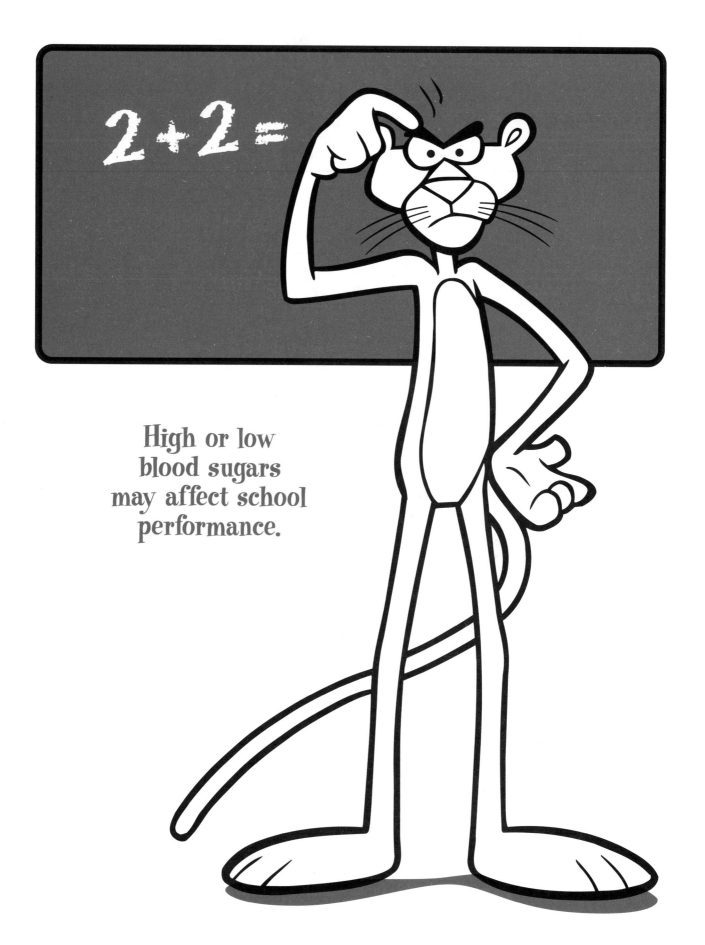

High or low blood sugars may affect school performance.

Chapter 18
Care of Children at Different Ages

Children of different ages are able to handle different tasks and responsibilities. These may vary from day to day and from week to week. This is true for diabetes-related tasks and non-diabetes tasks. Giving insulin injections for different aged children is discussed in Chapter 9. It can be helpful for family members to have an idea of what to expect at different ages. (See the Tables of age-responsibilities in the book, *"Understanding Diabetes,"* Chapter 18.) Goals for blood/CGM sugar levels and HbA1c values for children of different ages are included in Chapters 7 and 14.

BELOW AGE 8 YEARS

• Parents do all tasks.

• Children gradually learn to cooperate.

• Shots or boluses are often given after meals or snacks (rather than before) depending upon how reliably the child eats.

AGES 8-12 YEARS

• Children begin to give some of their own shots or assume some pump-related activities/responsibilities. A common mistake is to push for too much responsibility before the child is ready.

• Having a friend spend the night or staying at a friend's house often begins during this period. As the children are often very active and use more energy from staying up later than usual, it is best to reduce the insulin dose.

• At this age, fine motor control and the sense of accuracy needed to draw up the insulin develops.

• It is important to continue to check doses of insulin drawn by the child to make sure of accurate amounts. It is also important to check the blood/CGM glucose devices to review their readings.

• The idea of maintaining optimal sugar control to prevent later diabetes complications can initially be understood around ages 12 or 13 years.

AGES 13-18 YEARS

At this age, youth begin to have the ability to do all or most of their diabetes management, but are more successful if parents remain in a constant supportive role. They may need reminders for checking blood/CGM sugar levels or taking insulin 20 minutes prior to meals (see Chapter 8). One of the most difficult chores for many teens is writing the blood sugar values in a log book (or downloading meter or CGM results). It is important to do this, or trends in blood/CGM glucose values will be missed. Most glucose meters, pumps and CGMs can now be easily downloaded at home. Often the parents agree to do this (with the teen's OK). It is also a way for the parents to stay involved with the diabetes care and to step back in if blood/CGM glucose levels are not being evaluated. A decrease in the number of blood sugar checks per day is a major reason HbA1c levels tend to be higher in teenagers.

WHAT IS THE AGE WHEN SELF-CARE SHOULD HAPPEN?

- Children should be encouraged to assume self-care as they are able.

- There isn't a "magic" age when children should take over everything.

- If too much is expected too soon, feelings of failure and low self-esteem with poor diabetes self-care may result.

- **We believe that a supportive adult can be valuable for any person with diabetes, no matter the person's age.**

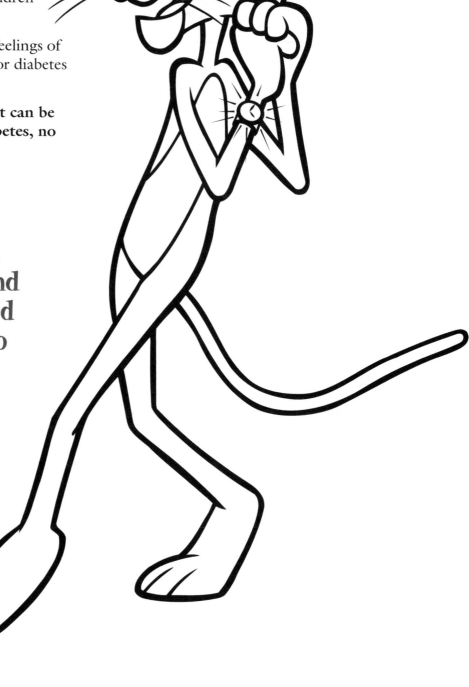

An alarm watch
may help to remind
a child of the need
for a snack, or to
give a shot or
bolus of insulin.

Children between the ages of 8-14
can begin to help manage their diabetes.

Chapter 19
Diabetes Management in the Toddler/Preschooler

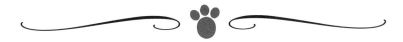

Chapter 18 deals with traits related and not-related to diabetes for different aged children including toddlers and preschoolers. Giving insulin shots to young children is discussed in Chapter 9. Although most of diabetes management is similar to that of older children, questions are often asked relating to insulin therapy.

BASAL-BOLUS INSULIN THERAPY
(also see Chapter 8)

When possible, basal-bolus insulin therapy, by injections or by an insulin pump, should be used in this age group. The use of NPH insulin is more apt to result in low blood/CGM glucose levels, particularly during the night. Very young children often need very small doses of insulin. This can be accomplished with half-unit pens or syringes, insulin pumps, and/or the use of diluted insulin. (U-20 or U-50 insulin instead of the standard U-100).

• **Injections**

The basal insulins are Lantus (or Basaglar), Levemir (occasionally given twice daily) and Tresiba (also called Degludec). They are usually given once daily – preferably in the morning in toddlers. Then if the insulin does not last a full 24 hours, insulin activity is less in the early morning hours when lows are worrisome. Some parents give the injection (often in the buttocks) while the child is still asleep.

The preferred bolus insulin is either Humalog, NovoLog or Aprida. In contrast to older children, the shot is sometimes given after the meal if eating is unpredictable in this age group. The dose can then be chosen after seeing what the child eats. Blood/CGM glucose levels will then be higher after meals in comparison to giving the bolus 20 minutes before the meal. This is a compromise to avoid hypoglycemia. Smaller (3ml) vials of Humalog can be ordered from pharmacies. (Tell the pharmacist the NDC number is 0002-7510-17.) There is also the HumaPen LUXURA® and the NovoPen Echo® which take 3 ml cartridges (of Humalog and NovoLog, respectively) and can give 0.5 unit doses. The Humalog Junior KwikPen is a disposable pen which can also give 0.5 unit doses. These are more accurate than using syringes.

• **Insulin Pumps**

About half of children in this age group in the U.S. are treated with insulin pumps. Advantages of insulin pumps (Chapter 28) are:

• Frequent shots are avoided

• More precise dosing is possible

• Variable basal rates throughout the day

• Ability to give multiple insulin doses with meals, snacks or high blood sugars. This means that a correction insulin dose plus a small amount of insulin for meal coverage can be given before the meal for an unpredictable appetite with the remainder given once the parents see what the child ate.

• Some pumps allow for remote dosing, so the child can receive an insulin bolus without interrupting playtime activity.

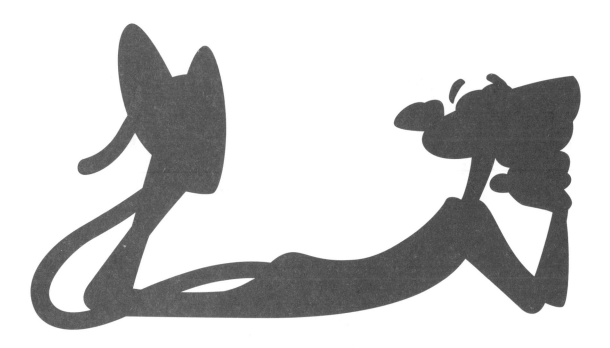

Several studies have shown that insulin pumps are safe in young children. The parents obviously do all of the pump management and must agree to wanting the pump for their child. For some parents, early pump use has been associated with more stress, although this usually lessens with time. The use of temporary basal rates or turning off the pump for periods of high activity or at the time of low blood/CGM glucose values can be advantageous (see Chapter 30). HbA1c levels may not always decrease with pump use in this age child. When used with a CGM, some pumps have the feature to stop insulin with a low CGM glucose value (see CGM below). The major reasons for pump use in this age group are safety and convenience.

SUGAR CONTROL

Our goal for fasting/before meal blood/CGM glucose levels (70-150 mg/dL or 3.9-8.3 mmol/L) is not as strict for this age group in comparison to older children. Likewise, the aim for bedtime/overnight glucose levels (100-180 mg/dL or 5.5-10.0 mmol/L) is not as strict for this age group in comparison to older children.

Our goals for sugar control are less stringent in young children for several reasons:

- Unpredictable eating

- Inconsistent physical activity

- Young children may not recognize or communicate hypoglycemic symptoms

- The brain is still developing and is especially sensitive to severe lows

- The risk for complication damage is low prior to puberty

- Small doses of insulin can have big effects on blood sugar levels in this age group

The ADA goals for blood/CGM sugar levels for all ages of youth are to be between 90-130 mg/dL (5.0-7.2 mmol/L) fasting/before meals, and 90-150 mg/dL (5.0-8.3 mmol/L) at bedtime/overnight. These levels are different than our recommendations (Chapter 7 and above) for this age group. There is now some evidence that high blood sugars and episodes of ketoacidosis can also have adverse effects on the developing brain (as with low blood sugar). This, along with aiming for lower HbA1c levels, is the reason for the ADA aiming for the lower sugar levels at bedtime and during the night in this age group.

The ADA goal for HbA1c levels is to have the value below 7.5 percent (<58 mmol/mol) in children and adolescents of all ages.

CONTINUOUS GLUCOSE MONITORS (CGM)

As with pumps, a CGM can be useful in this age group **when the family is ready** (see Chapter 29). This is particularly true for young children who cannot tell a parent when they are feeling high or low. The CGM provides convenience and comfort for the parents being able to see the glucose levels at any given time. For some devices, the CGM glucose levels can be transmitted "via the cloud" to a watch worn by the parent or to the parent's smart phone. This can give a parent who is away from the child a feeling of comfort for the child's safety.

Some blood sugar checks will still be necessary. They are necessary for daily calibrations of the CGM, and should always be checked with high and low glucose level alarms. The major drawback to CGM for young children is adequate locations for the insertions, especially if also using an insulin pump. The diabetes nurse educator can help to explore this issue. A major advantage is that when used with the Medtronic 530G or 630G insulin pump, the Threshold (low glucose) Suspend feature can help to prevent severe hypoglycemia (see Chapter 30). Because ketones (Chapter 15) form more rapidly in children ages nine years and below, it is wise to check the ketone level if the system has been turned off for the two hours maximum (to prevent hypoglycemia) or anytime the blood/CGM glucose level is above 300 mg/dL (>16.7 mmol/L).

ARTIFICIAL PANCREAS
(see Chapter 30)

The MiniMed/Medtronic 670G hybrid artificial pancreas was approved for use in people ages 14 years and older. It is not yet approved to use in younger children.

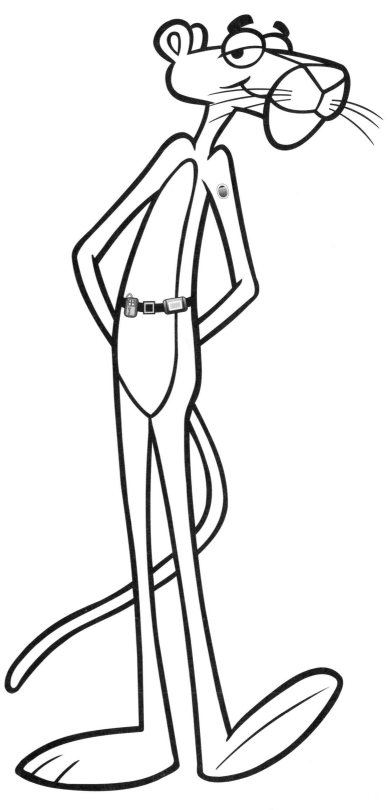

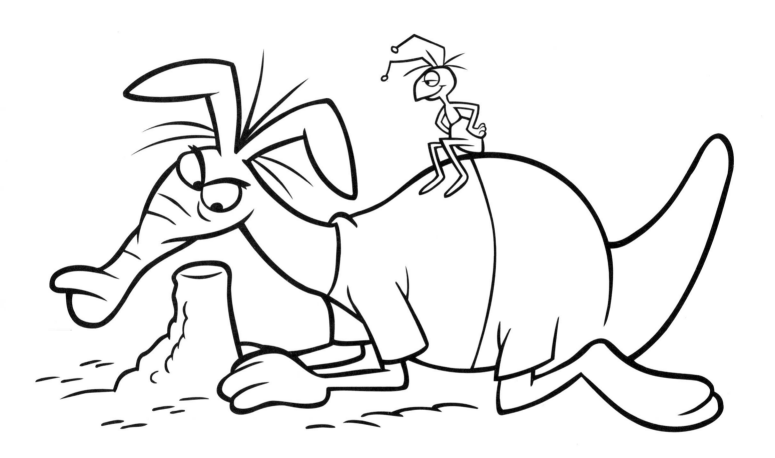

Chapter 20
Special Challenges of the Teen Years

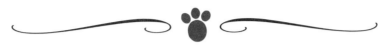

R
he teen years are a time when young people waver between wanting to be an independent adult and wanting to stay a dependent child. It is not surprising that they go back and forth when it comes to taking over the diabetes responsibilities. Many research studies now show that when parents stay involved in diabetes management, the diabetes will be in better control.

THE CHALLENGES

The teenage years are often the most difficult for having optimal sugar control (including an HbA1c value below 7.5 percent [58 mmol/mol]). And yet, they are important years in relation to an increased risk for diabetes complications.

If the number of blood sugar checks per day is reduced, or high CGM glucose levels are ignored, the HbA1c level will rise.

At least 30 (and preferably 60) minutes of physical activity daily is important, both for diabetes control and for a sense of well-being.

Growth and sex hormones are at high levels and interfere with insulin activity.

Insulin pumps, more frequent insulin shots or boluses, or use of the basal insulins, Lantus (Basaglar), Levemir or Tresiba (Degludec) rather than NPH insulin can help some teens. However, if meal and snack shots (or boluses for pumpers) are missed, the HbA1c value will increase.

Driving a car safely is very important beginning in the teen years. It is important to always check a blood/CGM glucose level before driving. Driving

with a low blood sugar can result in altered judgment and reactions that can be just as severe as if driving while drunk.

Diabetes is often not a priority to the teenager. Teenagers have special issues, including:

- **Struggle for independence**

- **Growth and body changes**

- **Self-identity**

- **Sports activities (see Chapter 13)**

- **Peer relationships**

- **Substance abuse (tobacco, alcohol, drugs, etc.)**

- **Sexuality (including anticipatory guidance for birth control and safe sex)**

- **Driving a car**

- **College**

- **Emotional changes**

- **Consistency**

Consistency is a key word in diabetes management. This may relate to food intake, exercise, stress, monitoring of blood/CGM glucose levels and timing of insulin shots/boluses. It is often hard for teens to be consistent.

These are all discussed in detail in the book, "Understanding Diabetes" (see order form in the back of this book).

Parents must:

- **Find ways to stay involved in diabetes management.** They can be helpful in keeping the log book, downloading meters, pumps or CGMs and in talking about insulin dosage.

- **Set and enforce reasonable expectations.**

- **Be available to help, but should try not to be overbearing or constantly nagging.** A supportive adult can be helpful for a person with diabetes, no matter the person's age.

- **Help with communication to the diabetes care-providers.** This may involve sending meter, pump or CGM data by email, fax or the cloud.

It is not surprising that diabetes is often referred to as a "disease of compromise."

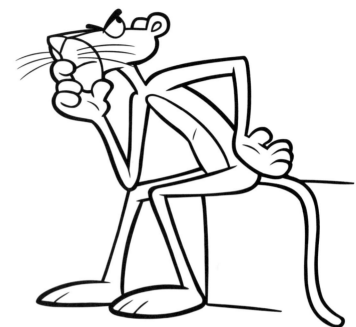

Teenagers have their own special challenges.

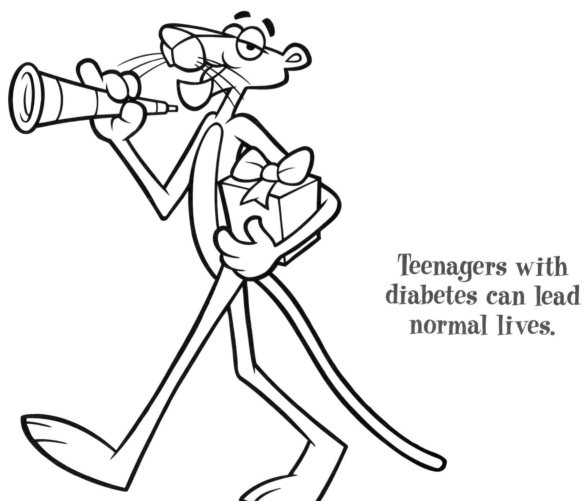

Teenagers with diabetes can lead normal lives.

Normal teen
activities can
provide much-needed
exercise.

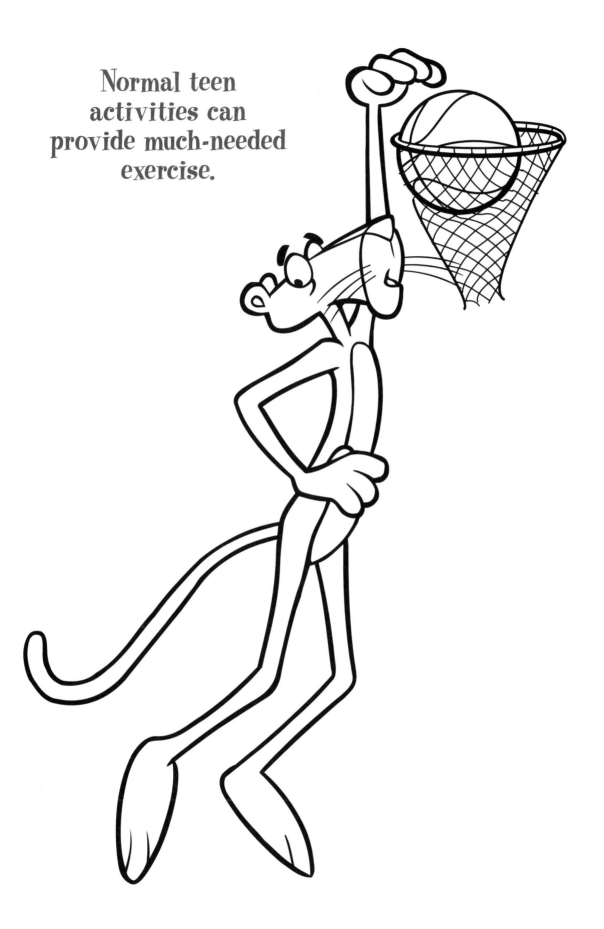

Clinic visits should be every three months for people with diabetes.

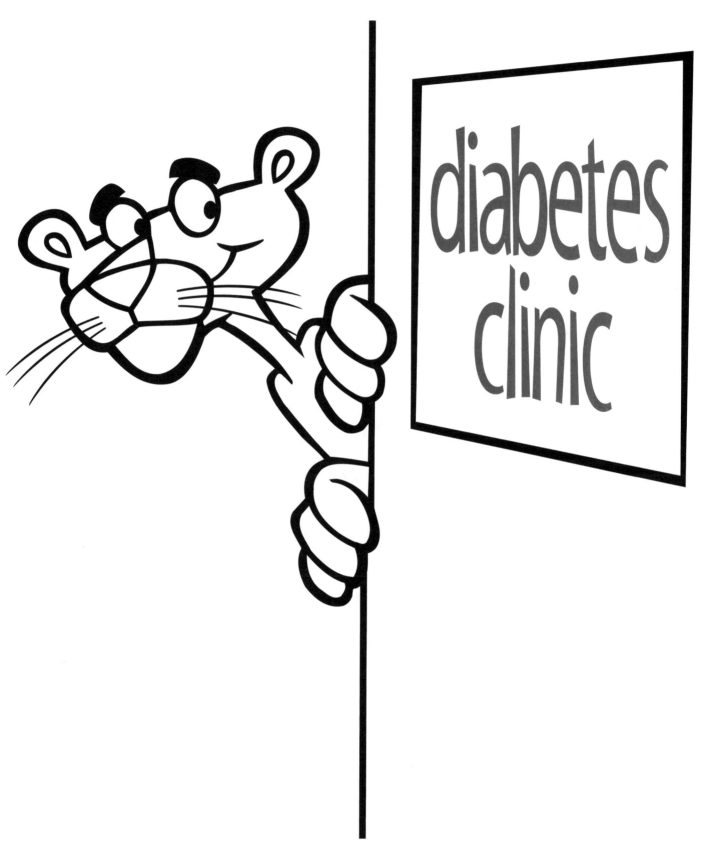

Chapter 21 – Outpatient Management, Support Groups, Education, and Standards of Care

Chapter 21
Outpatient Management, Support Groups, Education, and Standards of Care

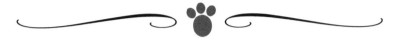

WHAT SHOULD HAPPEN AFTER A DIAGNOSIS OF DIABETES?

After initial education, people with diabetes should receive regular follow-up visits every three months. Diabetes education should continue for the patient and family at each visit.

The insulin doses may be changed during these visits. As children grow, they need more insulin. It is usually increased about one-half unit per pound of weight gained.

On the physical exam, thyroid size and eye changes are checked. Growth and other signs of sugar control are also checked. If blood/CGM glucose values have been high, the sugar may collect on the joint proteins and finger curvatures may result.

The HbA1c level (see Chapter 14) should be done every three months.

Initial screening for the eyes (eye exam) and kidneys (urine microalbumin) should be done for people who have had type 1 diabetes for five or more years, starting at age 10 years or at puberty, whichever is first (see Chapter 23). The frequency of repeat screening may vary depending on history of diabetes control.

For people with type 2 diabetes, the eye and kidney evaluations should be done at the time of diagnosis, and then yearly.

WHAT ELSE IS IMPORTANT?

Communication (fax, email, iCloud) of blood/CGM glucose values to the healthcare provider is often helpful (to receive suggestions for insulin dose changes).

Clinic visits by telemedicine are now available in some areas. These can be alternated with regular clinic visits so physical exam changes can be checked.

The families should let their diabetes provider or diabetes team know about any of the following:

- Any severe low blood sugar (hypoglycemic) reactions (with loss of consciousness or seizure)

- Frequent mild reactions

- Moderate or large urine ketones or blood ketones above 1.0 mmol/L

- Any planned surgery

- If at least half of the blood/CGM glucose values are not in the desired range for age (see Chapter 7)

SUPPORT GROUPS AND CONTINUING EDUCATION

Support groups, age-related group clinics, and special educational programs (Research Updates, Carb Counting Class, Pump or CGM classes, Grandparents Workshop, College-Bound Workshop, etc.) are available in many areas. The College Diabetes Network (website below) may be a helpful resource for youth adjusting to this new venture in life.

Special events (family workshops, bike trips, camps, a Halloween party, etc.) help children and families to learn more about diabetes. They also provide a chance to talk to others who have a family member with diabetes.

There are many excellent websites for people and families with diabetes. Some that we recommend are:

- www.barbaradaviscenter.org
- www.childrensdiabetesfoundation.org
- www.childrenwithdiabetes.com
- www.collegediabetesnetwork.org

- www.diabetes.org
- www.diatribe.org
- www.ispad.org
- www.jdrf.org
- www.myglu.org

STANDARDS OF CARE

The ADA (American Diabetes Association) "Standards of Care" are published each January as a supplement to the journal, *Diabetes Care*. The ISPAD guidelines are published in *Pediatric Diabetes*. The diabetes care team should be up to date on these standards. They can be found online.

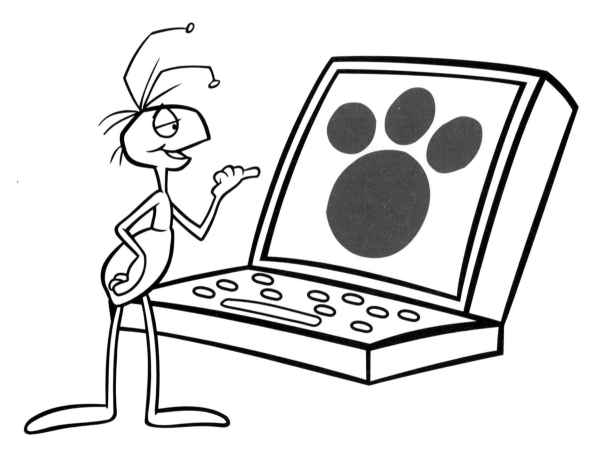

Faxing or emailing blood/CGM glucose values to the clinic between visits is very important. Mark your calendar for reminders to make follow-up visits every three months.

Mark your calendar to remind yourself of follow-up appointments every three months.

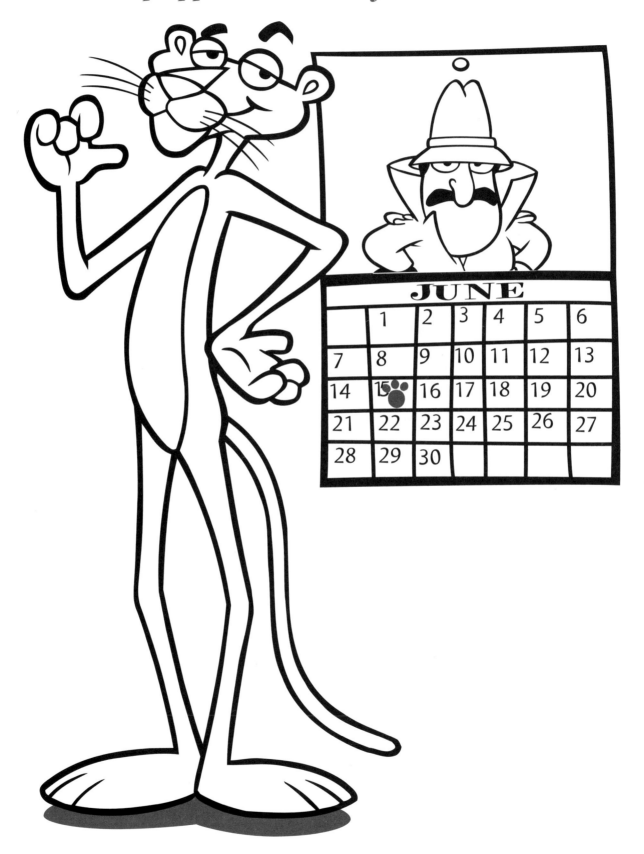

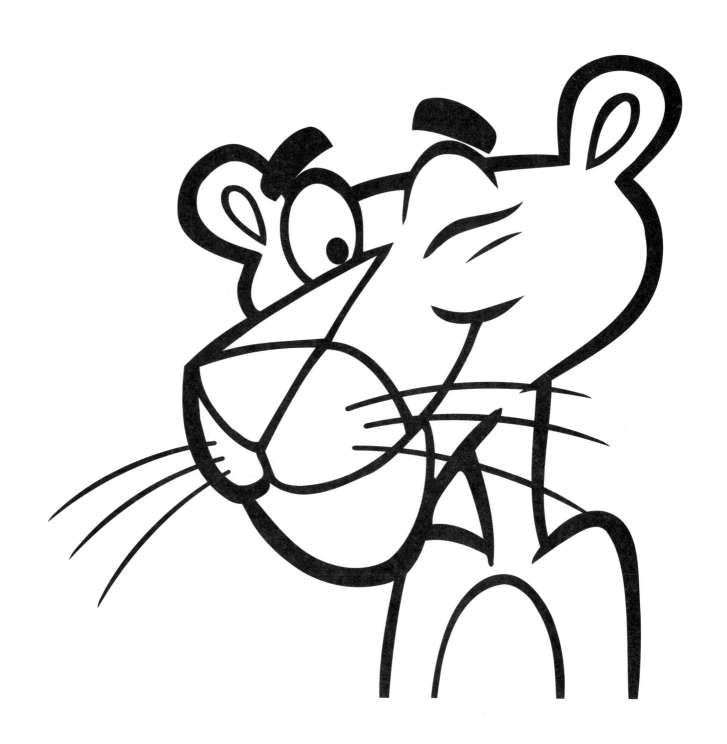

Ask if you need help
changing your dose!

Chapter 22
Adjusting Insulin Dosages

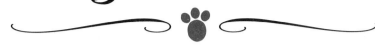

The FDA has approved the use of the Dexcom G5 and G6 and the FreeStyle Libre Flash continuous glucose monitors (CGM) for adjusting insulin dosages. Thus, this chapter will refer to adjustments done using finger-stick blood sugars or the CGM.

We encourage patients and families to learn to change the insulin doses on their own. Your diabetes care team is available if questions.

HOW AND WHEN SHOULD AN INSULIN DOSE BE CHANGED?

1. Looking at blood/CGM glucose patterns over the last week allows changes to be made.

It is necessary to know which insulin is acting at the time of the highs or lows in order to make the correct changes (see Figures in Chapter 8).

If using a CGM, families will develop their own practices for when to supplement the CGM glucose value with the finger-stick blood sugars. We generally recommend checking a finger-stick glucose with symptomatic or non-symptomatic low CGM sugars (e.g., CGM values ≤ 70 mg/dL or 3.9 mmol/L) or high CGM sugars (CGM values >300 mg/dL or 16.7 mmol/L). The CGM should not be used for insulin dosing if the person has recently received a medicine containing acetaminophen (e.g., Tylenol), because the CGM values may be falsely elevated. This is not a problem with the Dexcom G6.

If more than half of the blood/CGM glucose values at any time of the day are above the desired range for the age of the person (see Table in Chapter 7), the insulin dose acting at the time of the high sugar values should be increased. If

values are still high after three days, the dose can again be increased.

If changing basal rates on an insulin pump, remember that the insulin peaks in 90 minutes, so the dose must be increased or decreased an hour before the time of concern.

If there are more than two lows (e.g., below 70 mg/dL [3.9 mmol/L]) at one time of day, the insulin dose acting at that time should be decreased. If more lows occur, the dose can be decreased again.

2. The change in insulin dose will vary by age and "insulin sensitivity."

With small children, the change in dose may be by 0.05 to 0.5 units (smaller dosages are for changes in basal rates if using an insulin pump).

With older children and teens, the change in dose may be by one or two units.

Tables are given in the larger book, *"Understanding Diabetes"* (Chapter 22), for people wanting more detailed suggestions on changing insulin doses for high or low sugar values.

3. Correction (or sensitivity) factors are used to help adjust each insulin dose.

The correction (or sensitivity) factor refers to the number of units of insulin needed to correct or reduce a sugar value to a desired level.

The **correction factor** can be used to "correct" a high sugar value down to a **target blood/CGM glucose level** (e.g., 150 mg/dL [8.3 mmol/L] during the night and 120 mg/dL [6.7 mmol/L] during the day).

One example of a **correction factor** is to give one unit of insulin for every 50 mg/dL (2.8 mmol/L) of glucose above 150 mg/dL (8.3 mmol/L);

e.g., if the blood/CGM glucose level is 250 mg/dL (13.9 mmol/L), the correction factor is 2 units. Many teens and adults correct down to 120 mg/dL (6.7 mmol/L) or even 100 mg/dL (5.5 mmol/L) during the day. However, every person is different, and the correction factor should be adjusted to fit the individual.

If the correction factor being used is the correct dose, the sugar levels should be at target (corrected) after two to three hours. If this does not happen, the correction factor may need to be changed (e.g., to make correction more aggressive, you might change from 1 unit per 50 mg/dL [2.8 mmol/L] to 1 unit per 30 mg/dL [1.7 mmol/L]).

At bedtime, during the night, or before exercise, the correction dose is often reduced. This may be done by giving half of the calculated correction dose, by using a less aggressive correction factor (for example changing from 1 unit per 50 mg/dL [2.8 mmol/L] to1 unit per 100 mg/dL), or by using a higher target blood/CGM glucose level.

It is generally wise to wait at least two hours between correction insulin dosages to allow the rapid-acting insulin to have its effect.

Most people use a combination of a **correction factor** and an **insulin to carbohydrate (carb) ratio** (see Chapter 12) to determine the total dose of rapid-acting insulin before meals and snacks (see Table).

4. Changes in insulin dosages for food are discussed in Chapter 12.

Meal boluses are usually chosen based on the carbs to be eaten. The insulin to carbohydrate (I/C) ratios for different meals may be chosen by the dietitian or other diabetes team members.

One of the greatest deficiencies in diabetes management relates to a lack of blood/CGM sugar checks two and four hours after meals. The ADA recommends that all values be below 180 mg/dL (10 mmol/L). The use of a CGM can be a great aid in evaluating post-meal sugar levels.

The methods to increase or decrease I/C ratios are given in Chapter 12.

With the current rapid-acting insulins, giving the dose 20 minutes before eating is often very effective in lowering post-meal sugar levels (Chapter 8).

5. Changing dosage is similar for Lantus (Basaglar), Levemir or Tresiba (Degludec).

Adjustments are based primarily on the morning (fasting) sugar levels. Overnight blood sugar levels (or preferably CGM values) may help to understand the overnight trend.

Overnight data should be evaluated to determine if the basal insulin is peaking during the night or losing effect in the early morning. Other factors to be considered include exercise during the day or late-night meal boluses.

If blood sugars are rising overnight and morning blood sugars are consistently above the recommended values (see Chapter 7), basal doses are increased.

If blood sugars are dropping overnight and morning blood sugars are consistently below the recommended values, basal doses are decreased.

Dose changes for a young child may be by one half to one unit, and for older children (and teens) by one to two units.

Suggested waiting times between dose changes are 3-4 days unless follow-up sugar values are <70 or >300 mg/dL (<3.9 or >16.7 mmol/L). If this is the case, more frequent corrections can be made.

6. The use of "thinking" scales will aid in making insulin adjustments.

The insulin dose is figured by considering many factors, including:

- The blood/CGM glucose level
- If using CGM, the arrow and the direction of glucose change
- Illness (may increase needs)
- Any exercise that has been done or is planned (may decrease needs)
- Stress (may increase needs)
- Food to be eaten (use I/C ratio)
- Menses (may increase needs)

Families gradually learn to make insulin adjustments based on these factors.

It is VERY important to make insulin adjustments between visits if blood/CGM sugars are not in range half of the time or if low more than 10 percent of the time. Your diabetes care team is available if you have questions.

Table
Example of Determining an Insulin Dose

| Blood Sugar | | Correction Factor ** | Carbohydrates *** | | Total Units of Insulin |
mg/dL	mmol/L	Units of Insulin	Grams	Units of Insulin	
<150*	<8.3*	0	(15g)	1	1
151-200	8.4-11.1	1	(30g)	2	3
201-250	11.2-13.9	2	(45g)	3	5
251-300	14.0-16.7	3	(60g)	4	7
301-350	16.8-19.4	4	(75g)	5	9

* < means "less than"

** Assuming a correction factor of 1 unit of rapid-acting insulin per 50 mg/dL (2.8 mmol/L) above 150 mg/dL (8.3 mmol/L).

*** In this example, 1 unit of insulin is given for each 15g of carbs. The carbs are increased by 15g for each line in the Table.

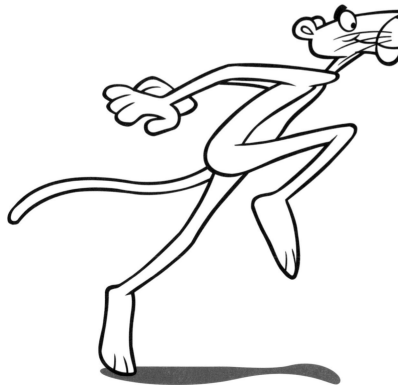

The insulin dose may need to change with the amount of food eaten or with sports activities ("thinking" scale).

Have your eyes checked regularly.

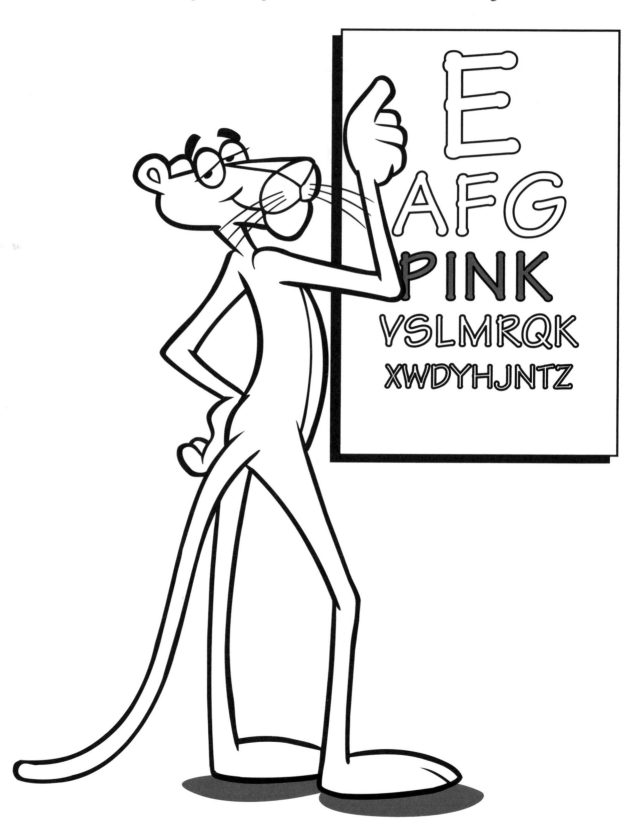

Chapter 23
Long-Term Complications of Diabetes

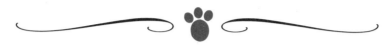

WHAT CAN REDUCE THE RISK OF DIABETES COMPLICATIONS?

- Optimal blood sugar control will reduce the risk for eye, kidney, nerve, and heart complications of diabetes by more than 50 percent, as shown by the DCCT (Chapter 14).

- Not smoking (or chewing) tobacco and avoiding smoke exposure is important.

- Other factors include treatment of elevated blood pressure or blood lipids (e.g., cholesterol). Even mild increases in blood pressure can damage the eyes and kidneys.

- Maintaining a healthy diet and weight (with exercise) is important.

- Optimal diabetes management (e.g., reaching HbA1c targets) reduces the risk of future complications.

HOW ARE COMPLICATIONS FOUND?

Small Blood Vessels (Eyes, Kidneys and Nerves)

- Regular eye exams (and especially photographs) by the eye doctor show if someone is developing eye damage.

- The urine microalbumin measurement shows if someone is getting early kidney damage at a time when it may still be reversible.

- Neuropathy screening is done as a foot exam during the clinic visit.

- According to the ADA, screening of the eyes (eye exam), kidneys (urine microalbumins) and nerves (foot exam) should be done annually for people who have had type 1 diabetes for five or more years, starting at age 10 years or at puberty, whichever is first.

- Some physicians now feel that if glucose control has been in range (e.g., HbA1c levels <8%), following the baseline exam, the above screening might be done every two years, rather than annually, prior to adulthood.

- People who have type 2 diabetes should have the eye and kidney evaluations done soon after diagnosis and then every year.

- Families may need to help remind the healthcare team that it is time to do the screening.

Large Blood Vessels (Including the Heart [Coronary] Blood Vessels)

- Heart attacks and other blood vessel diseases are a greater risk in adults with diabetes. Long-term optimal sugar control is important in prevention.

- Avoiding tobacco use and exposure is important for ALL people, but especially for people with diabetes.

- Maintenance of normal weight, blood pressure and cholesterol is also important in prevention.

- Cholesterol (lipid) levels should be screened at puberty, or sooner if there is a family history of high cholesterol.

- Adult diabetes clinics usually do special evaluations of the heart (EKGs) and blood vessels at regular intervals.

- Risk factors and aims for prevention are summarized in the Table.

TREATMENT

- The most important treatment of early complications involves improving sugar control. Maintaining normal weight, blood pressure, and cholesterol levels is also important.

- Treatment of early kidney damage is often helped by lowering blood pressure. A blood pressure medicine called an ACE-inhibitor is often used initially.

- If many eye changes are present, laser treatment to the back of the eye (retina) may help prevent more severe problems. This is almost never needed during the pre-adult years.

Table
Heart and Blood Vessel Risk Factors

Risk Factors	Aim for Prevention
glucose (sugar) control	HbA1c in recommended range for age
blood pressure	120/80 or below the 90th percentile for age
tobacco use	don't use, avoid exposure to second-hand smoke
elevated total cholesterol	below 200 mg/dL (5.2 mmol/L)
elevated LDL cholesterol	below 100 mg/dL (2.6 mmol/L)
elevated (fasting) triglyceride	below 150 mg/dL (1.7 mmol/L)

If any of the levels are elevated, it is important to discuss with your physician.

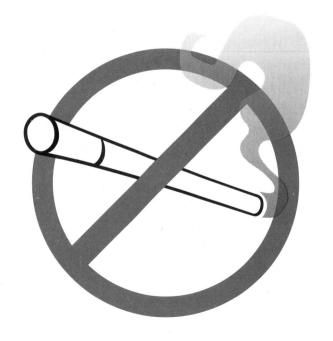

DO NOT SMOKE!
(or chew tobacco!)

Chapter 24
Associated Autoimmune Conditions of Type 1 Diabetes

Other autoimmune (self-allergy) diseases are also associated with type 1 diabetes. This is due to the inheritance of genes increasing the risk for autoimmunity (associated with both type 1 diabetes and these diseases). Three examples of autoimmune diseases seen more frequently in people with type 1 diabetes are discussed below.

THYROID PROBLEMS

Thyroid problems (like type 1 diabetes) are partly due to autoimmunity (see Chapter 3). Antibodies are made against the thyroid gland. About 1 in 10 people with diabetes need treatment with a daily thyroid hormone replacement pill for an underactive thyroid. More rarely, some people will have an overactive thyroid (1 in 100 people with diabetes).

We recommend careful examination of the thyroid gland with clinic visits. Laboratory evaluations should be done annually, particularly if the thyroid gland is enlarged or if there is any fall-off in growth. The TSH (Thyroid Stimulating Hormone) is the best laboratory value for screening. Some physicians also order a blood thyroid hormone level (T4 or free T4).

CELIAC DISEASE

This involves an allergy to the protein gluten, present in wheat, barley and rye. It occurs in approximately 1 of every 20 people with diabetes. There may be stomach complaints (pain, gas, diarrhea) or poor growth. Half of the people with celiac disease have no symptoms.

We recommend routine screening of all people with type 1 diabetes with the blood transglutaminase level (or other assays). If positive, it is important to work closely with GI (gastrointestinal) physicians. If the person with diabetes is positive, other family members should also be screened. The treatment is to remove all wheat, rye and barley products from the diet. Meeting with a dietitian is important. Websites for obtaining more information on celiac disease and foods to avoid are given in Chapter 24 of *"Understanding Diabetes,"* (see the back of the book for ordering).

ADRENAL DISORDERS

Autoimmunity against the adrenal gland (Addison's disease) can occur, but is quite rare (1 in 500 people with type 1 diabetes). Low adrenal gland function can be treated with hormone replacement pills and is important to diagnose if present. Cortisol, the hormone the body is unable to produce in Addison's disease, is especially important during body stress (e.g., surgery or a serious infection). Addison's disease can be life-threatening if untreated.

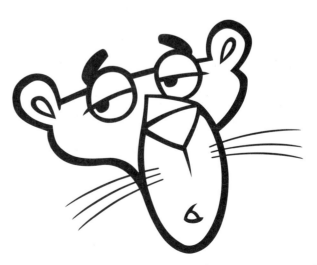

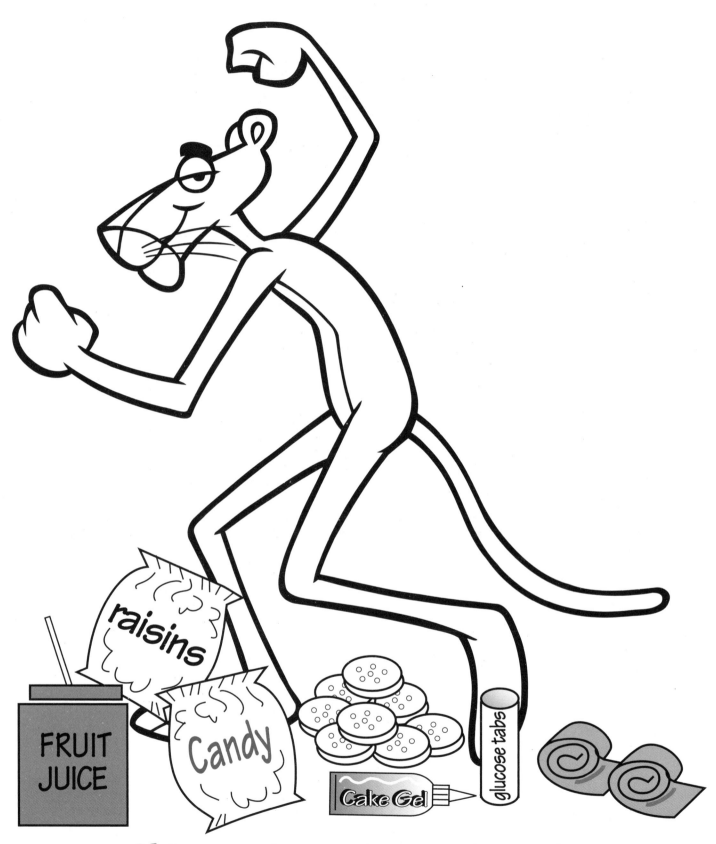

Make sure that you have snacks handy
at school in case you need them.

Chapter 25
The School or Work and Diabetes

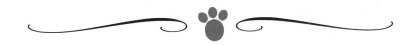

Most schools now require school health plans. Some schools use a basic "Standard of Care" for diabetes management for all youth (Table 1). The diabetes team then fills out the "Individualized Healthcare-Provider Order for Student with Diabetes," depending on whether using insulin injections (Table 2) or an insulin pump (Table 3). Alternatively, a combined Standards of Care plus Healthcare-Provider Orders or an Individualized Health Plan (IHP) is available in Chapter 25 of *"Understanding Diabetes"* (see reference 2 at end of Table 1). You are welcome to copy the Tables in this chapter and in Chapter 25 in *"Understanding Diabetes."*

The parents must also provide supplies for the school. Some children keep a separate meter and strips at the school. Others bring their home meter and supplies in their backpack. Some children will use the Dexcom G5 Continuous Glucose Monitor (CGM), which has been approved by the FDA for choosing insulin dosages (see below). It should not be used if the person has received a medicine containing acetaminophen (e.g., Tylenol). The Dexcom G6 is not affected by acetaminophen. Others may be using the MiniMed/Medtronic 670G Artificial Pancreas System, which delivers insulin, and increases, decreases or stops insulin administration automatically, based on CGM glucose levels (see Chapter 30).

Other forms that you may want to copy from *"Understanding Diabetes"* (Chapter 25) are:

1) Individualized Health Plan – School Nurse Checklist

2) Insulin Pumps in the School Setting

3) Continuous Glucose Monitoring (CGM) in the School

4) School Supply Checklist

WHAT CAN HAPPEN AT SCHOOL?

- **Low blood/CGM sugar (hypoglycemia, insulin reaction)** is the most likely emergency to occur at school. Treatment is reviewed in Table 1. If a child leaves the classroom while having a low blood sugar, they **MUST** have someone with them. It may be helpful for the family to copy and review the Table in Chapter 6 on mild, moderate and severe reactions with the school personnel. Supplies for treating lows will also need to be provided by the family.

- **High blood/CGM sugar levels** may also occur at school, particularly with stress, illness, menses, overeating or lack of exercise. If the blood/CGM sugar level is above 300 mg/dL (16.7 mmol/L) on two checks (≈ 1 hour apart), the urine or blood ketones need to be checked. When the blood/CGM sugar is high, it is generally necessary to go to the bathroom more frequently, which must be allowed. Treatment for high blood sugar and high blood or urine ketones is reviewed in Table 1. *If urine ketones are moderate or large, or blood ketones are above 1.0 mmol/L, we generally recommend that the parents be called to come and take the student home in order to be treated and monitored more closely.*

WORK

People with diabetes must have all necessary diabetes supplies and snacks readily available at work. The American Disabilities Act states that employers must provide "reasonable accommodations to allow a person with diabetes to safely and successfully perform their job." Friends, family and some co-workers and/or supervisors need to know about the diabetes and, at a minimum, what to do in case help is needed for a low blood sugar. An emergency plan to provide essential details is included at the end of Chapter 14 in the book *"Management of Diabetes in Adults"* (see ordering material in the back of this book).

Forms in this chapter are available for download at: **www.barbaradaviscenter.org**. Search under "Patient Care" tab for "Clinical Resources" link.

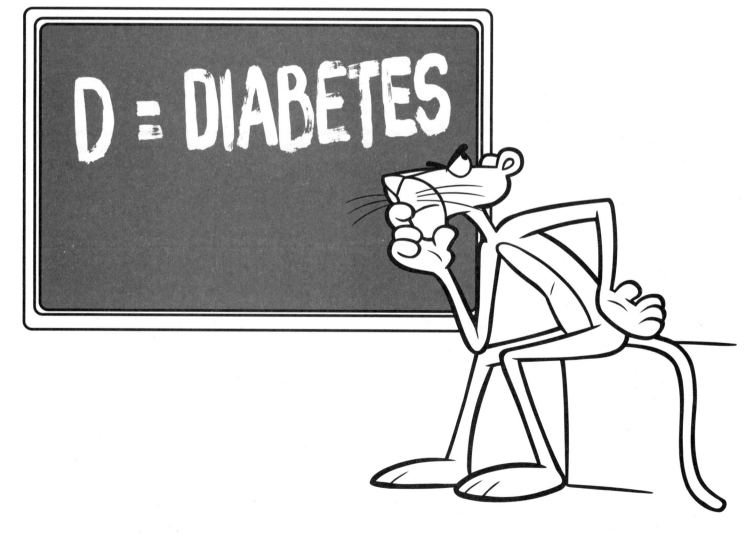

Table 1
Standards of Care for Diabetes Management in the School Setting & Licensed Child Care Facilities

modified from *www.coloradokidswithdiabetes.com*

These are general standards of care for students with Type 1 Diabetes to be used in conjunction with the Provider Orders (Table 2 or 3). The student's diabetes healthcare-provider may indicate exceptions to these standards on the student's individual orders.

1. **Communication:** To facilitate appropriate execution of the Diabetes Healthcare-Provider's orders and to ensure safety of the student, the school nurse/Child Care Nurse Consultant (CCNC) will have authorization to exchange health information with the healthcare-provider to assist in developing, updating and carrying out the Individualized Healthcare Plans (IHP). The school nurse/CCNC has permission for care coordination per signed diabetes healthcare-provider orders, which aligns with both Health Insurance Portability and Accountability Act (HIPAA) and Family Educational Rights and Privacy Act (FERPA) regulations. The student's healthcare plan is developed by the school nurse/CCNC in collaboration with the parent/guardian(s) and healthcare-provider. Communication of blood glucose readings and coordination of care between student, school nurse/CCNC, healthcare-providers, school staff/teachers and/or parents may include a variety of options (e.g., cell phone applications, web-based applications, email, or texting). Shared data plans and/or Wi-Fi will need to be provided by the parents if necessary for cellphone service and/or remote site monitoring.

2. **Diabetes Healthcare-Provider Orders:** Orders should be obtained annually for the start of each school year and ongoing as needed or annually/ongoing based on enrollment into a child care facility. If ongoing changes to the insulin dosing is a total of +/- 3 units per dose outside the current orders on file, then parents should contact the diabetes healthcare-provider for new orders to reflect these changes. Additional school or district specific medication forms are unnecessary unless they contain additional information not specified for this student's diabetes care.

3. **Monitoring Blood Glucose:** *The student's healthcare-provider should indicate individualized blood glucose target ranges on the student's individual order (e.g., Table 2 or 3).*

   Standard Target Ranges Before Meals: The student's target ranges are indicated by the diabetes care-provider. If the target range is not indicated, please refer to Table 2 or 3, or to the ADA recommendation of a pre-meal range of 90-130mg/dL (per reference 1 below).

   (Symbols used: < = less than; > = greater than; ~ = approximately)

   The frequency of routine blood glucose monitoring should take into consideration the student's schedule and participation in classroom learning/activities. Too frequent routine glucose monitoring may impact learning and school participation. On average, a student would have routine glucose monitoring one to three times during the school day unless otherwise indicated on orders.

4. **Hypoglycemia (low sugar level, insulin reaction)**

   - Student should be treated *immediately (i.e., classroom, playground)* if symptomatic or if blood glucose is below target range. If the student needs to go to the Health Office, the student **must** be accompanied by a responsible person.

   - A student with hypoglycemia should be treated first, prior to notifying parents.

   - Check finger-stick blood glucose with a glucose meter if student reports feeling low. If no blood glucose meter is available, assume that blood sugar is low and treat accordingly.

   - **Mild symptoms:** If blood glucose is **below** target range and/or student is symptomatic (e.g., shaky, hungry, pale), treat with ~15g fast-acting carbohydrate (e.g., juice, glucose tabs, etc.) (if student <5 y.o. give ~7.5g of fast-acting carbohydrate unless otherwise indicated). **Retest** in 10-15 minutes. Repeat 15g (7.5g for <5y.o.) fast-acting carbohydrate every 10-15 minutes until **within** target range. When blood glucose is **within** target range, follow with 15g snack (protein and carbohy-drate) or lunch/meal (unless otherwise indicated on orders). Do not give insulin for this snack unless indicated (see Note below).

   - **Moderate symptoms:** (e.g., not thinking clearly) Check blood glucose; if unable to drink juice, administer glucose gel. Re-treat as above until within target range. If unable to administer, and intranasal glucagon (3 mg) is available, it may be used. Follow with snack or lunch (see Note below).

- **Severe symptoms:** may include seizures, unconsciousness, unable or unwilling to take juice or gel: If BG meter is readily available, check blood glucose level prior to treating to confirm hypoglycemia. If on insulin pump, turn pump off or disconnect tubing.

  ○ **Administer glucagon and call 911**

    - Glucagon dose is indicated on the Provider orders. Doses of 0.5 ml (<12 years) or 1.0 ml (12 years or older) are encouraged for accurate administration in the school setting. If intranasal glucagon is available, it may be used (3 mg) instead of injected glucagon.

    - Trained personnel should be available for administration of injected glucagon.

Note:

For Injections: Do not give insulin for carbohydrates given to <u>treat</u> low blood glucose. The School Nurse/CCNC should discuss with the parent whether the student is to be given insulin for snacks immediately following hypoglycemia (school nurse/CCNC to make note in Table 2 below).

If at lunchtime, after blood glucose is within target range, send the student to lunch and give insulin after eating, based on the *recovered* blood glucose level and grams of carbs, unless otherwise indicated on orders.

For Insulin Pumps: Don't enter the carbohydrate grams in pump that were given to treat the low blood glucose. The school nurse/CCNC should discuss with the parent whether the student is to be given an insulin bolus for snacks immediately following hypoglycemia (School nurse/CCNC to note in Table 3 below).

If at lunchtime, after blood glucose is within target range, send the student to lunch. After eating, enter *recovered* blood glucose level and grams of carbs eaten into pump and use the pump calculator to determine amount of insulin to be given, unless otherwise indicated on orders.

Notify Parents after student has been treated for hypoglycemia.

If more information related to hypoglycemia is desired, refer to Chapter 6 in this book, or to reference 2 below.

5. **Hyperglycemia (high sugar levels)**

No pump (see 7, Insulin Management below for insulin instructions):

- If BG is above the target range, and it has been over 3 hours since the last dose of insulin, provide insulin for BG correction as indicated in the orders below. If at lunchtime, include the insulin to cover the meal carbohydrates, as in the orders below.

- The school nurse should take into consideration upcoming activities, including PE, lunch dosing, walking home, afterschool activities, etc., when giving insulin corrections for high BG (for both injections and pumps). *If the correction factor is not available, or there is not a sliding scale for insulin dosage, contact the Diabetes Care-Provider for a one-time order.*

- If BG >300 mg/dL (16.7 mmol/L) after two consecutive checks (≈ 2 hours apart), <u>or</u> illness, such as nausea/vomiting, TEST KETONES. Check one: blood ⃝ urine ⃝ ketones.

- If no method to check ketones is available, call parents to come to do the ketone check or to take student home to monitor and treat.

- If ketones are below moderate in urine or 1.0 mmol/L in blood, student may require insulin in-jection. First, contact parent. If parents are not available, call diabetes care-provider for further instructions.

- Recommend student be released to parents when ketones are moderate or large in urine or >1.0 mmol/L in blood, or if student has symptoms of illness (e.g., nausea, vomiting), in order to be treated and monitored more closely by parent/guardian.

- If ketones present, provide water and keep student from exercise.

With Pump (see 8, Pump Management below for insulin instructions):

⊙ If BG is above the target range, and it has been over 3 hours since the last dose of insulin, provide insulin for BG correction as indicated in the orders below. If at lunchtime, include the insulin to cover the meal carbohydrates, as in the orders below.

⊙ The school nurse should take into consideration upcoming activities, including PE, lunch dosing, walking home, afterschool activities, etc., when giving insulin corrections for high BG (for both injections and pumps). *If the correction factor is not available, or there is not a sliding scale for insulin dosage, contact the Diabetes Care-Provider for a one-time order.*

⊙ If BG >300 mg/dL (16.7 mmol/L) after two consecutive checks (≈ 2 hours apart), or illness, such as nausea/vomiting, TEST KETONES. Check one: ☐ blood ☐ urine ☐ ketones.

- If no method to check ketones is available, call parents to come to do the ketone check or to take student home to monitor and treat.

- If ketones are below moderate in urine or 1.0 mmol/L in blood, student may require insulin injection. First, contact parent. If parents are not available, call diabetes care-provider for further instructions.

- Recommend student be released to parents when ketones are moderate or large in urine or >1.0 mmol/L in blood, **or** if student has symptoms of illness (e.g., nausea, vomiting), in order to be treated and monitored more closely by parent/guardian.

- If ketones present, provide water and keep student from exercise.

⊙ **Potential pump malfunction:** The concern for a student on a pump with prolonged hyperglycemia is the possibility of blocked insulin tubing and the risk of going into Diabetic Ketoacidosis (DKA). This can happen after 2 or 3 hours without insulin. Unlicensed assistive personnel should contact school nurse for further instructions regarding insulin by injection or new infusion set by parent or independent student.

Note: For all students (pump or no pump), the school nurse/CCNC and parent should contact the healthcare-provider for insulin dose adjustments if hyperglycemia occurs frequently.

6. **Exercise and School Attendance (for students on insulin injections and/or pump):**

Student Symptoms & BG level	Ketone Level	Exercise	Stay in School
>300mg/dL first time, no symptoms	None	Yes	Yes
>300mg/dL – 2 consecutive times (over 2 hours apart), no symptoms	None	Yes	Yes
>300mg/dL no symptoms	Trace-Small	Yes*	Yes
>300mg/dL **with symptoms**	None	No	No
>300mg/dL, with or without symptoms and urine ketones are moderate-large or blood ketones >1.0	Urine: Moderate-Large or Blood ketones >1.0	No	No
>300, 2 consecutive times, no symptoms	Unable to check ketones	No	No †
>300, with symptoms	Unable to check ketones	No	No

*School Nurse/CCNC should determine if type of exercise is appropriate (e.g., weather conditions – exercise may not be appropriate, student's hydration status, school's ability to monitor symptoms during exercise, etc.).
Note: *always check blood glucose and/or ketones before exercise if the student is not feeling well.*
† Parent may bring ketone-checking equipment to school to determine status.

7. **Insulin Management (injections or pumps):**

- Fast-acting insulins are interchangeable (e.g., Humalog, NovoLog, Apidra) unless student is allergic to a certain brand or otherwise indicated.

- The parent and/or unlicensed assistive personnel should contact the school nurse/CCNC if changes in insulin dosing are called for.

- In the school setting, fast-acting insulin is ideally given (injection or pump) approximately 5-20 minutes prior to lunchtime, unless otherwise indicated. Since it is difficult to determine precisely when the student will actually eat their meal at school due to varying factors, fast-acting insulin is not given earlier than 20 minutes to avoid an episode of hypoglycemia. The two-digit rule may be used, if recommended by your care-provider. This is a rule using the first 2 digits of the blood glucose to how much in advance to give insulin prior to a meal, e.g., if blood glucose is 200 then give insulin 20 minutes (maximum time interval) before eating, or if 150 give 15 minutes before eating. If blood glucose is below 70 mg/dL, wait to give insulin until after the meal.

- Refer to student's individualized orders for snack dosing.
- After 28 days, opened vials/cartridges/pens of insulin will begin to lose their potency and be susceptible to bacteria contamination; therefore, the insulin should no longer be used in the school setting.
- Please check with parents to see whether they would like the used insulin to be returned to them or discarded.

8. Pump Management

- The computerized features/calculator of pump should be used for insulin boluses.
- **All** blood glucose values and carbohydrate grams to be eaten (with the exception of treatment for hypoglycemia) must be entered into the pump for delivery of pump-recommended boluses.
- Parents/guardians are responsible for ensuring all pump settings align with orders.
- The pump bolus calculator rarely should be overridden (e.g., in dosing changes). Encourage parents to follow up with their healthcare-provider for insulin pump dose adjustments if frequent overrides are being requested.
- Delegated staff should always get approval from their school nurse to override pump insulin calculations.

9. Continuous Glucose Monitors (CGM)

- CGM systems use a tiny sensor inserted under the skin to monitor glucose levels (ongoing or short term) in interstitial fluid. Level sometimes varies from BG values; if so, always accept the BG result. The CGM is calibrated to the student using a finger-stick glucose reading when readings are stable, approximately two or three times/day, typically outside of school. Parents/independent students are responsible for changing sensor/site. Calibration may need to occur in school if prompted by CGM, and should ideally occur when the blood glucose levels are stable (not rising or falling rapidly).
- In the school setting, delegated school staff should respond to low and high BG alarms rather than to the constantly fluctuating trends and numbers.
- The FDA has approved use of the Dexcom G5 and G6 and the FreeStyle Libre Flash CGM glucose values to make insulin treatment decisions without needing to test finger-stick blood glucose (BG) values. If more information is needed, please refer to reference 3 or 4 below.
- For all other CGMs, always confirm a CGM reading with a finger-stick glucose reading prior to insulin administration. (Do not enter sensor reading into pump for insulin calculation.)
- Remote monitoring of the CGM in the school setting is generally not required, as the student is usually adult-supervised by trained school staff and frequent routine BG monitoring is scheduled as indicated. It is not the responsibility of school personnel to monitor the CGM readings. However, in certain unique cases (e.g., preschool age, non-verbal, impaired cognition, severe hypoglycemia unawareness) monitoring/remote monitoring may be appropriate, and the school nurse/CCNC, along with the Section 504 Team, will determine this need based on the student's individual unique need(s). When determined appropriate, the school nurse/CCNC will indicate these accommodations on a Section 504 plan and the IHP.
- Reasonable use of the CGM in the school setting will foster the student's ability to recognize when they have symptoms of hypo/hyperglycemia.
- Parents will set the alarms and notify the school nurse/CCNC of the parameters. Alarms should be used sparingly and only for safety, to avoid unnecessary disruption of the student's school activities (i.e., set alarms only for glucose levels that require an immediate action/response).

10. Advanced Pump Technologies in the school setting – *These are recently FDA approved:*

- **Medtronic MiniMed 530/630 G Pump:** Threshold Suspend/Suspend on Low *is a feature on Medtronic pump and CGM systems which automatically suspends* insulin delivery if the sensor detects a low glucose level. When triggered, the pump turns itself off, sounds a siren alarm, and requires the user to choose between leaving the basal insulin off or restarting it. A finger-stick BG should be done and the appropriate treatment for low glucose initiated if the BG is truly low. If no action is taken, the pump continues to alarm and remains off for up to 2 hours or until the user chooses to resume insulin delivery. During this automatic suspension time, no bolus insulin can be given.

- **Medtronic MiniMed 670 G pump with hybrid artificial pancreas technology:** This has four levels of operation including 1) **basal insulin delivery**, 2) **Suspend on Low**, 3) **Suspend Before Low** mode which automatically stops insulin 30 minutes before reaching the student's pre-selected low limits, then automatically restarts (without alerts) insulin when levels recover and 4) **Auto Mode** which is a considered a closed-loop system. It automatically adjusts basal insulin delivery every 5 minutes based on CGM sugar levels to keep student in target range around the clock. **The system is called hybrid because an insulin bolus for food (as discussed in: 7, Insulin Management, see above) must still be given by the person or by the School Nurse/CCNC.** For more information on insulin pumps, contact the Diabetes Resource Nurse for your area, your Medtronic pump representative, or reference 3 or 4 below.

11. **Self-Care Management:**
- Ability level to be determined by school nurse/CCNC & parent unless Provider indicates otherwise (see Table 2 or 3).
- All students, regardless of age or expertise, may require immediate assistance with hypoglycemia and/or illness.

12. **Student with private duty nurses:** *The Standards of Care* may be individualized or exempt at the discretion of the parents and/or healthcare-provider and per any agreement with the school district.

13. Table 2 (for student using injections) or Table 3 (for student using insulin pump) will also be completed.

NOTE: School and Child Care nurses can determine their individual scope of practice regarding new diabetes treatment therapies and/or diabetes care practices at https://www.colorado.gov/pacific/dora/Nursing_laws.

REFERENCES:

1. American Diabetes Association (January, 2018): Standards of Medical Care in Diabetes, Diabetes Care 41 (Supplement 1). www.diabetes.org/diabetescare
2. Chase, H.P., & Maahs, D.M., (2015). *Understanding Diabetes (13th Ed)*. Denver, CO. Paros Press. Available at 303-863-1200, or www.childrensdiabetesfoundation.org.
3. Chase, H.P., & Messer, L., (2017). *Understanding Insulin Pumps & Continuous Glucose Monitors (3rd Ed.)*. Denver, CO. Paros Press. Available at 303-863-1200, or www.childrensdiabetesfoundation.org.
4. Colorado Kids with Diabetes Care and Prevention Collaborative, www.coloradokidswithdiabetes.org

I agree with this standard of care.

Signed: _____ Date: _____
　　　　　　　　Parent(s)

This Table may be copied as desired.

Table 2
Individualized Health Plan (IHP) for Student with Diabetes Using Injections

Student: _____DOB:_____ School: _____ Grade: _____

Physician: _____Phone:_____

Diabetes Educator:_____

Parent name(s) and phone number(s) _____

_____

WHEN TO CHECK BLOOD GLUCOSE: *For provision of student safety while limiting disruption to learning*

☑ **Always for signs & symptoms of low/high blood glucose, when does not feel well and/or behavior concerns**

- ☐ Before School Program   ☐ Before Snack   ☐ Mid-morning   ☐ After School Program/Extracurricular Activity
- ☐ Before Lunch   ☐ After Lunch   ☐ Recess   ☐ Before PE   ☐ After PE
- ☐ School Dismissal   ☐ Before riding bus/walking home   ☐ 2 hrs after correction
- ☐ Other: _____

TARGET RANGE – Blood Glucose: ☐ _____ to ☐ _____

- ☐ (suggested for <6 y.o.)   ☐ (suggested for 6 – 17 y.o)   ☐ (suggested for >17 y.o.)
  70-150 mg/dL (3.9-8.3 mmol/L)   70-130 mg/dL (3.9-7.2 mmol/L)   70-130 mg/dL (3.9-7.2 mmol/L)

Notification to Parents if blood glucose is less than _____ or greater than: _____

The following devices may be used for blood glucose in place of finger stick:
(See instructions in Table 1, Standards of Care, for instructions on when these may be used.)

☐ Dexcom G5/G6   ☐ Freestyle Libre   ☐ Other:_____

The following two sections are discussed in more detail in the Standards of Care (Table 1)

HYPOGLYCEMIA: See Standards of Care (Table 1) for more information.

Student should be accompanied to health office if symptomatic or BG below _____.

- If symptomatic but glucose meter not available, treat as indicated for mild symptoms below.
- If blood glucose in range _____ – _____ but symptomatic, treat with 10 to 15 gm carbohydrate snack.
- If mild symptoms (e.g., shaky, hungry, pale) test BG and if below _____, treat with juice, glucose tabs, etc. every 10-15 min until BG above _____. Then give 10-15 gm carb snack or give lunch.
- Do not give insulin for glucose used to treat hypoglycemia. If at lunchtime, wait to give meal insulin until after the meal.
- If moderate symptoms (e.g., not thinking clearly), they may be unable to drink independently. Test BG and administer sugar drink or glucose gel. If unable to administer, may use intranasal glucagon (3 mg) if available. Re-test every 15 minutes until BG above _____. Then give a snack that includes 10-15 gm carbs, or lunch.
- If severe reaction (seizure, unconscious), test BG and administer glucagon _____units (__cc/mL) IM into thigh; or, if available, intranasal spray glucagon (3 mg) may be used instead. ***Give nothing by mouth! CALL 911 AND PARENT.***
- Other: _____

HYPERGLYCEMIA AND KETONE TESTING:

- If BG is above the target range, and it has been over 3 hours since the last dose of insulin, provide insulin for BG correction as indicated in the orders below. If at lunchtime, include the insulin to cover the meal carbohydrates, as in the orders below.

- The school nurse should take into consideration upcoming activities, including PE, lunch dosing, walking home, after-school activities, etc., when giving insulin corrections for high BG (for both injections and pumps). *If the correction factor is not available, or there is not a sliding scale for insulin dosage, contact the Diabetes Care-Provider for a one-time order.*

  - If BG greater than 300 mg/dL (16.7 mmol/L) after two consecutive checks (≈ 2 hours apart), 5 illness, such as nausea/vomiting, TEST KETONES. Check one: ☐ blood ☐ urine

  - If no method to check ketones is available, call parents to come to do the ketone check or to take student home to monitor and treat.

  - If ketones are below moderate in urine or 1.0 mmol/L in blood, student may require insulin injection. First, contact parent. If parents are not available, call diabetes care-provider for further instructions.

  - Recommend student be released to parents when ketones are moderate or large in urine or above 1.0 mmol/L in blood, **or** if student has symptoms of illness (e.g., nausea, vomiting), in order to be treated and monitored more closely by parent/guardian.

  - If ketones present, provide water and keep student from exercise.

- Other: _____

CGM

- Parents will set alarms for CGMs sparingly to avoid unnecessary disruption of school activities (i.e., set alarms for blood glucose levels that require immediate action). Parents will notify school nurse of the parameters (e.g., alarm set for BG lower than 70 mg/dL [3.9 mmol/L]).

Alarms set for this student : Lower limit _____   High glucose alarm:_____

Insulin Dosing Orders (Insulin-to-Carb Ratios Plus the High BG Correction):

Carbohydrates and Insulin Dosage Injection at: ☐ Breakfast   ☐ Snack   ☐ Lunch   ☐ Other:

Bolus for carbohydrates should occur: ☐ Approximately 20 minutes Prior to lunch/snack

☐ Immediately before lunch/snack   ☐ Immediately after lunch/snack   ☐ Split ½ before lunch & ½ after lunch

☐ Other: _____

Insulin to Carbohydrate (I/C) ratio dose (to use if food to be consumed):

Time	Carbohydrate ratio
_____ to _____	1 unit of insulin per _____ grams of carbohydrate
_____ to _____	1 unit of insulin per _____ grams of carbohydrate
_____ to _____	1 unit of insulin per _____ grams of carbohydrate
_____ to _____	1 unit of insulin per _____ grams of carbohydrate

☐ Parent/guardian authorized to increase or decrease insulin to carb ratio 1 unit +/- 5 grams of carbohydrates

Sensitivity/Correction Factor:

Give _____ units of insulin for every _____ mg/dL (mmol/L) above the Target Blood Glucose Range (see above).

Time	Correction Dose
_____ to _____	Give _____ units of insulin for every _____ above _____.
_____ to _____	Give _____ units of insulin for every _____ above _____.
_____ to _____	Give _____ units of insulin for every _____ above _____.
_____ to _____	Give _____ units of insulin for every _____ above _____.

OTHER INSULIN/MEDICATIONS:

Basal Insulins: _____ units of _____ given at _____   Administered ☐ Home ☐ School

Intermediate Insulins (e.g., NPH): _____ units of _____ given at _____   Administered ☐ Home ☐ School

Oral Medications: _____ mg of _____ given at _____   Administered ☐ Home ☐ School

Student's Self Care: (Ability level determined by school nurse and parent with input by healthcare-provider)

Independently monitors blood/CGM glucose   ☐ Yes ☐ No

Independently treats mild hypoglycemia   ☐ Yes ☐ No

Independently counts carbohydrates   ☐ Yes ☐ No

Independently tests urine/blood ketones   ☐ Yes ☐ No

Self-injects with verification of dosage   ☐ Yes ☐ No   Injections to be done by trained staff.

Additional Information/Comments:

Signatures:

My signature below provides authorization for the written orders above and exchange of health information to assist the school nurse. I understand that all procedures will be implemented in accordance with state laws and regulations and may be performed by unlicensed designated school personnel under the training and supervision provided by the school nurse. This order is for a maximum of one year.

Physician: _____Date: _____

Parent: _____Date: _____

School Nurse: _____Date: _____

Table 3
Individualized Health Plan (IHP) for Student with Diabetes Using Insulin Pump

Student: _____ DOB: _____ School: _____ Grade: _____

Physician: _____ Phone: _____

Diabetes Educator: _____

Parent name(s) and phone number(s) _____

_____

WHEN TO CHECK BLOOD GLUCOSE: *For provision of student safety while limiting disruption to learning*

☑ **Always for signs & symptoms of low/high blood glucose, when does not feel well and/or behavior concerns**

☐ Before School Program ☐ Before Snack ☐ Mid-morning ☐ After School Program/Extracurricular Activity

☐ Before Lunch ☐ After Lunch ☐ Recess ☐ Before PE ☐ After PE

☐ School Dismissal ☐ Before riding bus/walking home ☐ 2 hrs after correction

☐ Other: _____

TARGET RANGE – Blood Glucose: ☐ _____ to ☐ _____

☐ (suggested for <6 y.o.) ☐ (suggested for 6 – 17 y.o) ☐ (suggested for >17 y.o.)
70-150 mg/dL (3.9-8.3 mmol/L) 70-130 mg/dL (3.9-7.2 mmol/L) 70-130 mg/dL (3.9-7.2 mmol/L)

Notification to Parents if blood glucose is less than _____ or greater than: _____

The following devices may be used for blood glucose in place of finger stick:
(See instructions in Table 1, Standards of Care, for instructions on when these may be used.)

☐ Dexcom G5/G6 ☐ Freestyle Libre ☐ Other: _____

The following two sections are discussed in more detail in the Standards of Care (Table 1)

HYPOGLYCEMIA: See Standards of Care (Table 1) for more information.

Student should be accompanied to health office if symptomatic or BG below _____.

- If symptomatic but glucose meter not available, treat as indicated for mild symptoms below.

- If blood glucose in range _____ – _____ but symptomatic, treat with 10 to 15 gm carbohydrate snack.

- If mild symptoms (e.g., shaky, hungry, pale) test BG and if below _____, treat with juice, glucose tabs, etc. every 10-15 min until BG above _____. Then give 10-15 gm carb snack or give lunch.

- Do not give insulin for glucose used to treat hypoglycemia. If at lunchtime, wait to give meal insulin until after the meal.

- If moderate symptoms (e.g., not thinking clearly), they may be unable to drink independently. Test BG and administer sugar drink or glucose gel. If unable to administer, may use intranasal glucagon (3 mg) if available. Re-test every 15 minutes until BG above _____. Then give a snack that includes 10-15 gm carbs, or lunch.

- If severe reaction (seizure, unconscious), test BG and administer glucagon _____units (__cc/mL) IM into thigh; or, if available, intranasal spray glucagon (3 mg) may be used instead. *Give nothing by mouth! SUSPEND OR DISCONNECT PUMP. CALL 911 AND PARENT.*

- Other: _____

HYPERGLYCEMIA AND KETONE TESTING: (see Pump Insulin Dosing orders below):

- If BG is above the target range, and it has been over 3 hours since the last dose of insulin, provide insulin for BG correction as indicated in the orders below. If at lunchtime, include the insulin to cover the meal carbohydrates, as in the orders below.

- The school nurse should take into consideration upcoming activities, including PE, lunch dosing, walking home, after-school activities, etc., when giving insulin corrections for high BG (for both injections and pumps). *If the correction factor is not available, or there is not a sliding scale for insulin dosage, contact the Diabetes Care-Provider for a one-time order.*

    - If BG greater than 300 mg/dL (16.7 mmol/L) after two consecutive checks (≈ 2 hours apart), 5 illness, such as nausea/vomiting, TEST KETONES. Check one: ☐ blood ☐ urine

    - If no method to check ketones is available, call parents to come to do the ketone check or to take student home to monitor and treat.

    - If ketones are below moderate in urine or 1.0 mmol/L in blood, student may require insulin injection. First, contact parent. If parents are not available, call diabetes care-provider for further instructions.

    - Recommend student be released to parents when ketones are moderate or large in urine or above 1.0 mmol/L in blood, **or** if student has symptoms of illness (e.g., nausea, vomiting), in order to be treated and monitored more closely by parent/guardian.

    - If ketones present, provide water and keep student from exercise.

- *Potential pump malfunction:* The concern for a student on a pump with prolonged hyperglycemia is the possibility of blocked insulin tubing and the risk of going into Diabetic Ketoacidosis (DKA). This can happen after 2 or 3 hours without insulin. Unlicensed assistive personnel should contact school nurse or diabetes care-provider for further instructions regarding insulin by injection or new infusion set by parent or independent student.

- Other: _____

PUMP INSULIN DOSING ORDERS (Insulin-to-Carb Ratios Plus the High BG Correction): Enter BG and approximate grams of carbs to be eaten. A suggested insulin dose will appear. Then just press "accept" or "enter" to give bolus.

Insulin Pump: (Type of pump: _____; type of insulin in pump:_____)

- Pump settings are established by the student's healthcare-provider and should not be changed by the school staff. All setting changes to be made at home or by student authorized to provide self-care.

- Parents will set alarms for pumps and CGMs sparingly to avoid unnecessary disruption of school activities (i.e., set alarms for blood glucose levels that require immediate action). Parents will notify school nurse of the parameters (e.g., alarm set for BG below 70 mg/dL [3.9 mmol/L]).

- Alarms set for this student : Lower limit _____   High glucose alarm:_____

Correction Bolus:

- Provide Correction bolus per pump calculator. Corrections should not be given more frequently than every 2 hours. The BG level should be entered into the pump for calculation of pump-calculated correction bolus. Press "enter" or "accept" to give the bolus.

Sensitivity/Correction Factor: (The correction factor below is to be used only if pump is not working.)

Time	Correction Dose
_____ to _____	Give _____ units of insulin for every _____ above _____ .
_____ to _____	Give _____ units of insulin for every _____ above _____ .
_____ to _____	Give _____ units of insulin for every _____ above _____ .
_____ to _____	Give _____ units of insulin for every _____ above _____ .

Carbohydrates and Insulin Dosage per pump at: ☐ **Breakfast**   ☐ **Snack**   ☐ **Lunch**   ☐ **Other:**

Bolus for carbohydrates should occur: ☐ Approximately 20 minutes Prior to lunch/snack

☐ Immediately before lunch/snack   ☐ Immediately after lunch/snack   ☐ Split ½ before lunch & ½ after lunch

☐ Other: _____

Insulin to Carbohydrate (I/C) ratio dose (to use if food to be consumed; typically programmed into pump):

Time	Carbohydrate ratio
_____ to _____	1 unit of insulin per _____ grams of carbohydrate
_____ to _____	1 unit of insulin per _____ grams of carbohydrate
_____ to _____	1 unit of insulin per _____ grams of carbohydrate
_____ to _____	1 unit of insulin per _____ grams of carbohydrate

☐ Parent/guardian authorized to increase or decrease insulin to carb ratio 1 unit +/- 5 grams of carbohydrates

---

Insulin Pump Basal Rates: (The pump gives these doses automatically and they are included only for information.)

Start Time:	Units per Hour:

PUMP MALFUNCTIONS: Disconnect pump when malfunctioning (usually due to plugged pump tubing).

- Check ketones if needed (see Hyperglycemia and Ketone Testing section above)
- If ketones are moderate/large (urine) or greater than 1.0 mmol/L (blood), follow instructions in Hyperglycemia and Ketone Testing section above.
- If pump calculator is operational, the insulin dosing should be calculated by using the pump bolus calculator and then insulin given by injection.
- If pump calculator is not operational, give insulin by injection using Insulin to Carbohydrate Ratio and Correction Factor above.

Student's Self Care: (Ability level determined by school nurse and parent with input by healthcare-provider)

Independently monitors blood/CGM glucose	☐ Yes	☐ No	
Independently treats mild hypoglycemia	☐ Yes	☐ No	
Independently counts carbohydrates	☐ Yes	☐ No	
Independently tests urine/blood ketones	☐ Yes	☐ No	
Independently manages pump boluses	☐ Yes	☐ No	Needs assistance with pump management.
Self-injects with verification of dosage	☐ Yes	☐ No	Injections to be done by trained staff.
Independently inserts infusion sets	☐ Yes	☐ No	Needs assistance.
Troubleshoots all alarms	☐ Yes	☐ No	Needs assistance with pump management.

Additional Information/Comments:

Signatures:

My signature below provides authorization for the written orders above and exchange of health information to assist the school nurse. I understand that all procedures will be implemented in accordance with state laws and regulations and may be performed by unlicensed designated school personnel under the training and supervision provided by the school nurse. This order is for a maximum of one year.

Physician: _____Date: _____

Parent: _____Date: _____

School Nurse: _____Date: _____

Chapter 26
Child-sitters, Grandparents and Diabetes

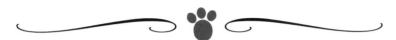

It is important for parents to feel that their child is safe with caregivers other than the parents. It is also important for these caregivers to feel confident that they can provide diabetes care.

WHAT DO THEY NEED TO KNOW?

How much training is needed will depend upon the amount of time the child will be with the caregiver and the age of the child.

All caregivers need:

- Some information about signs of low blood sugar and how to treat. Being prepared for a low blood sugar is essential.

- Some basic instruction on foods and diabetes. A handout is in this chapter which can be cut out or copied for the caregiver.

- Emergency phone numbers in case the parents cannot be reached. This helps everyone feel better.

- To know how to give shots or boluses by pump, how to check blood/GCM glucose levels, when to check for urine or blood ketones and other more detailed information if the parents are to be away for a longer time period. It may be easier to learn to give the insulin(s) using an insulin pen.

- An extra supply of insulin, etc. (in case a bottle is dropped and broken). An extra glucagon kit (and knowing where it is kept) is also helpful.

Attending a "Grandparent Workshop" or other workshop can help to teach the grandparents, baby-sitters or other caregivers about diabetes.

- It is important for the child and the grandparents to continue to have a close relationship.

- It can also help to remove any fears about giving shots or treating low blood sugars.

Caregivers may wish to join the parents at initial education classes or at the time of clinic visits. They are always welcome.

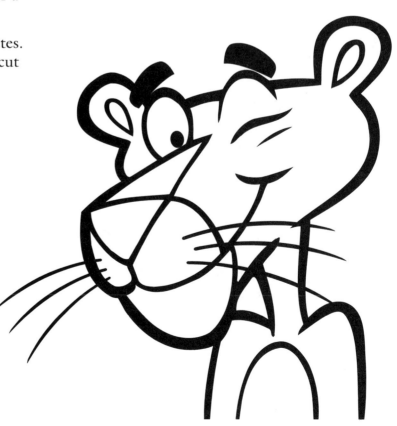

INFORMATION FOR THE SITTER OR GRANDPARENT

Our child, _____, has diabetes.

Children with diabetes are generally normal and healthy. In a child who has diabetes, sugar cannot be used by the body because the pancreas no longer makes the hormone insulin. Because of this, daily insulin injections or an insulin pump are needed. Diabetes is not contagious. Caring for a child with diabetes does require a small amount of extra knowledge.

LOW BLOOD SUGAR

The only emergency that could come on quickly is LOW BLOOD SUGAR (otherwise known as "hypoglycemia" or an "insulin reaction"). This can occur if the child gets more exercise than usual or does not eat as much as usual. *The warning signs of low blood sugar vary (see Chapter 6) but may include any of the following:*

1. Hunger
2. Paleness, sweating, shaking
3. Eyes appear glassy, dilated or "big" pupils
4. Pale or flushed face
5. Personality changes such as crying, being unreasonable or stubborn
6. Headaches
7. Inattention, drowsiness, sleepiness at an unusual time
8. Weakness, irritability, confusion
9. Speech and coordination changes
10. If not treated, loss of consciousness and/or seizure

The signs our child usually has are: _____

_____

_____

Blood Sugar: It is ideal to check the blood sugar with hypoglycemia, if this is possible (even if the child has a continuous glucose monitor [CGM] device). It takes 10-15 minutes for the blood sugar to increase after taking liquids with sugar. Thus, the blood sugar can even be done after taking sugar. If it is not convenient to check the blood sugar, go ahead with treatment anyway.

Treatment: Give SUGAR (preferably in a liquid form) to help the blood sugar rise.

You may give any of the following:
1. One-half cup of soft drink that contains sugar – **NOT a diet pop**
2. Three or four glucose tablets, sugar packets or cubes
3. One-half cup of fruit juice
4. LIFE-SAVERS (FIVE or SIX pieces) or other candy that has a low choking risk
5. One-half tube of Insta-Glucose or cake decorating gel (see below)

COPY AS NEEDED

We usually treat reactions with: _____

_____

If the child is having a low blood sugar and he/she refuses to eat or has difficulty eating, give Insta-Glucose, cake decorating gel (1/2 tube) or other sugar source. Put the Insta-Glucose, a little bit at a time, between the cheeks (lips) and the gums and tell the child to swallow. If he/she can't swallow, lay the child down and turn the head to the side so the sugar (glucose) doesn't cause choking. You can help the sugar solution absorb by massaging the child's cheek.

Severe reactions (unconscious, seizure) are rare. If trained in giving, glucagon can be given by injection or, if available, by intranasal spray. Either works in 10-20 minutes (see Chapter 6).

If a low blood sugar (insulin reaction) or other problems occur, please call:

1. Parent: _____ at: _____

2. _____ at: _____

3. _____ at: _____

MEALS, SNACKS AND INSULIN

The child must have meals and snacks on time. The schedule is as follows:

	Time	Food to Give	Insulin to Give
Breakfast			
Snack			
Lunch			
Snack			
Supper			
Snack			

Sometimes young children will not eat meals and snacks at exactly the time suggested. If this happens, DON'T PANIC! Set the food within the child's reach (in front of the TV set often works) and leave him/her alone. If the food hasn't been eaten in 10 minutes, give a friendly reminder. Allow about 30 minutes for meals.

BLOOD SUGARS

It may be necessary to check the blood sugar (Chapter 7) or ketones (Chapter 5).

The supplies we use are: _____

The supplies are kept: _____

Please record the results of any blood sugars or urine ketones.

Time: _____ Result: _____

C O P Y   A S   N E E D E D

INSULIN PUMPS

Many young children now receive their insulin via an insulin pump. The depth of knowledge about pumps will depend on the time of stay. At a minimum, you must be able to turn the pump off (or disconnect the tubing) with a low blood sugar and to turn it back on when the blood sugar rises. Also, if a very high blood sugar occurs (± ketones), a new infusion set may be needed (or a temporary shot of insulin). Parents often stay in close contact (when possible) to help advise.

If the stay is to be more than a few hours, it may be necessary to know how to approximate the amount of carbohydrates (carbs) to be eaten and to enter the value in the pump. If the blood sugar meter does not communicate automatically with the pump, the blood sugar value will also need to be entered. An insulin dose is then suggested by the pump and only needs to be accepted.

SIDE TRIPS

Please be sure that if the child is away from home, with you or with friends, extra snacks and a source of sugar are taken along, as well as a way to check blood sugar.

OTHER CONCERNS: *Concerns that we have are:*

_____

_____

_____

_____

_____

_____

_____

_____

_____

_____

If there are any questions or if our child does not feel well or vomits, please call us or the other people listed above. Thank you.

COPY AS NEEDED

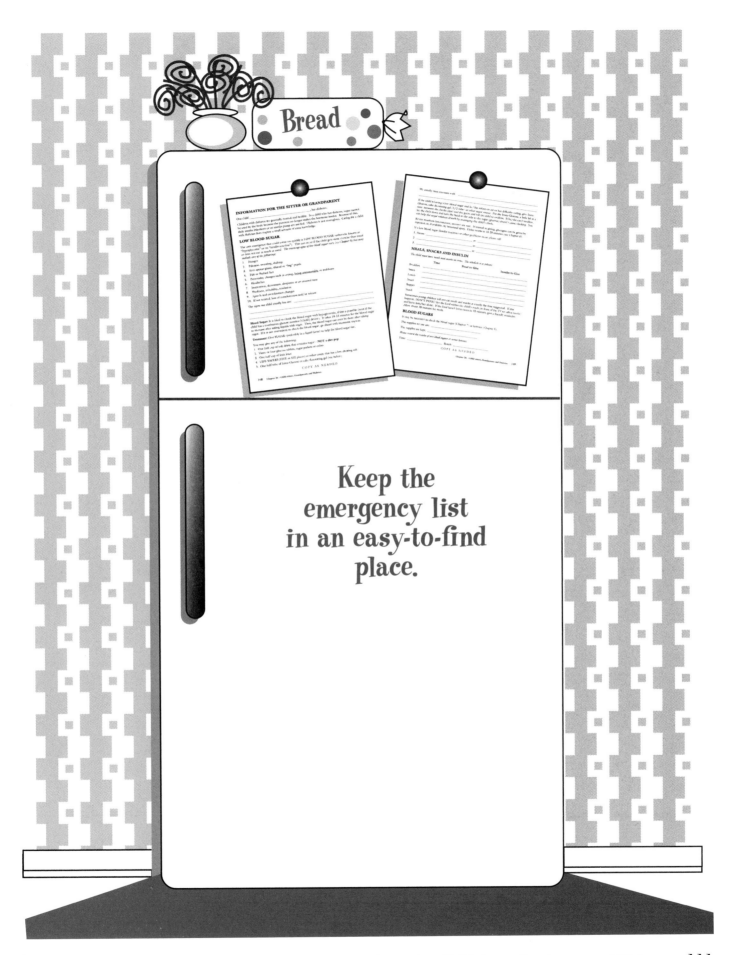

Keep the
emergency list
in an easy-to-find
place.

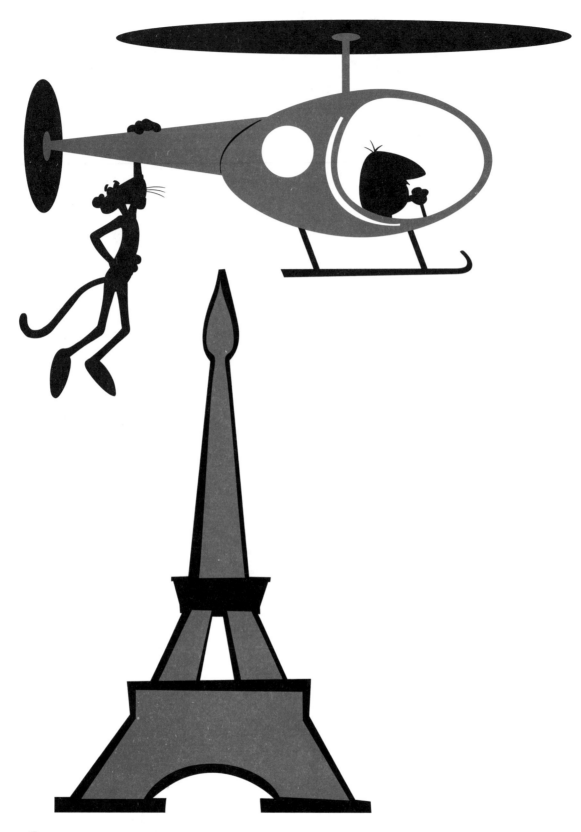

Special planning is important for vacations.
Be prepared for anything when
you're planning to camp or vacation.

Chapter 27
Vacations and Camp

WHEN TRAVELING, WHAT SHOULD PLANNING INCLUDE?

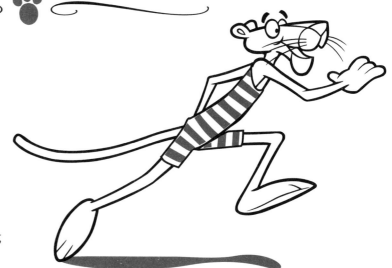

- Insulin, blood sugar and ketone strips, glucagon and CGM sensors must be kept in a plastic bag in a cooler if traveling by car. All will spoil if they get above 90° F (32° C) or if they freeze.

- If the meter has been in a cold place, it should be brought to room temperature before doing a blood sugar.

- Car travel may result in higher blood/CGM glucose levels due to less activity. Extra basal and bolus insulin is sometimes given. Those with insulin pumps can use increased temporary basal rates.

- Remember to take supplies for measuring ketones.

- Insulin and all critical supplies should always be available and hand-carried on airplanes, not packed in checked luggage. This ensures the insulin is not lost or subject to extreme heat or cold.

- It is important with airplane travel to have a vial of insulin with the pre-printed pharmacy label on the outside of the box. The glucagon should also be left in its original container. There have been no problems with taking insulin, insulin pumps or other diabetes supplies through security. Insulin pumps and continuous glucose monitors (CGM) should be worn and not put on the x-ray belt or exposed to a body scanner, as electronic components can be altered by x-ray. A travel letter from the diabetes doctor may also be required (including his/her phone number).

- Extras of everything should be carried by a second person when possible, in case one carry-on is lost.

- Extra snacks (sugar [dextrose] tablets, granola bars, etc.) should be carried, in case food is late or not available.

- Time changes within the U.S. are usually not a problem, but they must be considered if going overseas. Call your doctor or nurse for help with insulin adjustments if needed. For insulin pumps, the time in the pump should just be reset to the new time zone. This is important as your basal rates should match your sleep/wake cycle where you are and not left set to your home time zone.

- If traveling by plane and wearing an insulin pump, the high altitude sometimes causes pressure and extra insulin to be administered. Temporary basal rates or discontinuing insulin during pressure changes (take-off and landing) is sometimes needed (maximum of two hours).

- If activity is to be increased during vacations, such as playing at the beach, fishing, hiking, going to an amusement park, etc., the insulin dose should be decreased.

113

CAMP

Diabetes camp is often the first chance for a child and parents to show they can survive without each other. Most camps have doctors and nurses present so that the children are safe. Getting to know other children with diabetes who are of a similar age can be very helpful. Most of all, camp should be fun!

If going to a non-diabetes camp (or school camp/outdoor lab):

• It is essential the camp nurse and cabin counselor know about diabetes (low blood sugars and what to do, high blood sugars and what to do, illness and what to do, etc.).

• Insulin changes for camp will need to be made by the child's diabetes doctor or nurse. Insulin dosages are often reduced by 20 or 30 percent – particularly for the first few days at camp.

• All diabetes supplies will need to be provided by the family.

• Phone numbers need to be provided to report blood/CGM sugar values if needed and to receive insulin dose changes, as well as for any emergency.

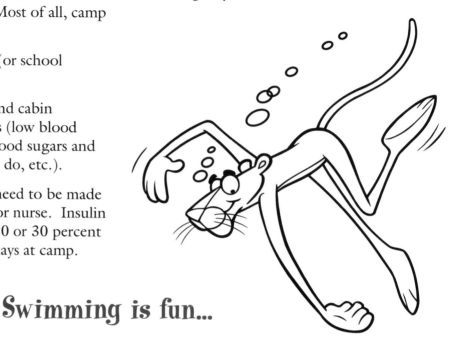

Swimming is fun...

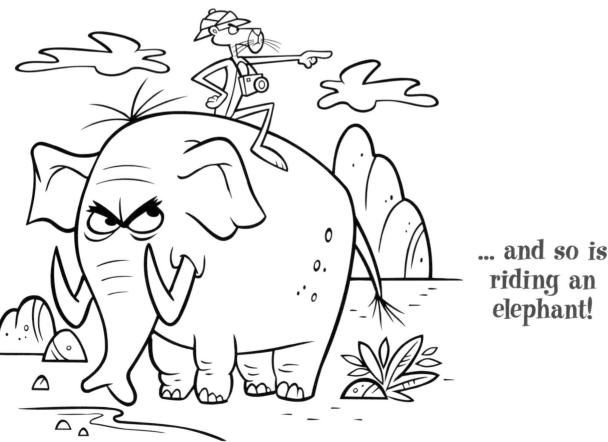

... and so is riding an elephant!

Chapter 28
Insulin Pumps

THE PUMP

An insulin pump is a micro-computer (the size of a pager) worn externally that constantly provides insulin. Only rapid-acting insulin is used in pumps. Pumps have become more popular in recent years. Advantages and disadvantages of pumps are discussed in Chapter 28 in the larger book, *"Understanding Diabetes."* In addition, there is a book all about pumps and other diabetes technologies, *"Understanding Insulin Pumps, Continuous Glucose Monitors and the Artificial Pancreas"* (see "Ordering Materials" in the back of this book). After reading one or both of these resources, the family may wish to discuss possible pump use and selection with their diabetes care-providers. If insurance will cover a continuous glucose monitor (CGM; Chapter 29), it may be helpful to order this at the same time. Both the insulin pump and CGM are essential parts of the artificial pancreas.

HOW IS INSULIN GIVEN BY THE PUMP?

The **basal** insulin dose provides a preset amount of short-acting insulin each hour. This can be changed at any time to fit the person's needs. This takes the place of long-acting insulins such as Lantus (Basaglar), Levemir or Tresiba (Degludec).

A **bolus** insulin dose is entered/given by the person wearing the pump (or by an adult) each time food is to be eaten or if a high blood/CGM glucose level is found.

WHAT IS INVOLVED WHEN STARTING ON A PUMP?

- The first week (and for some, the first month) is the most difficult as the system is learned.

- At least four blood sugars per day, or use of a CGM, must routinely be done prior to starting a pump.

- Carbohydrate counting (see Chapter 12) and correction factors (Chapter 22) are used to determine bolus doses.

- All pumps are now "smart pumps" and have insulin-to-carbohydrate (I/C) ratios and correction factors programmed into them (or into a linking meter) by the physician and family. Then, when a blood/CGM sugar level and/or grams of carbohydrate to be eaten are entered, the pump suggests an appropriate insulin dose. This dose can be given as suggested or it can be changed.

- Bolus dosages for food are best taken 20 minutes before eating (unless the blood/CGM glucose level is low).

- When young children are treated with a pump, the parents are responsible for counting carbohydrates and giving the bolus insulin doses (see Chapters 12 and 19).

- Basal and bolus insulin doses are individualized for each person. The physician usually suggests initial basal rates, insulin to carbohydrate ratios and correction factors. These can then be altered as needed for different times of the day.

- Alternate basal rate patterns can also be entered for special situations (extreme exercise, illness, menstrual cycle, etc.).

- Close contact with the healthcare-providers is essential.

- Our experience shows that children do well using an insulin pump if they and their parents are highly motivated.

- *The person with diabetes must be ready for the pump. It must not be just the parents (other than for very young children).*

FOUR DIFFICULTIES SEEN WITH INSULIN PUMP USE

- Forgetting to give bolus insulin doses will result in a high HbA1c level.

- Not doing at least four blood sugars per day (or consistently wearing a CGM) may lead to a high HbA1c level.

- The cannula (tube) coming out from under the skin, or the tube kinking, will interrupt insulin delivery and cause blood/CGM glucose levels to rise rapidly. Ketones begin to form after three hours with no insulin (or after two hours in children aged nine years or younger).

- Some people do not want to have a device constantly attached.

FOUR ADVANTAGES OF INSULIN PUMP USE

- **Insulin boluses are readily available when needed, and multiple boluses can be given without needing multiple needle pokes.**

- Insulin dosages can be finely tuned for different periods of the day.

- Insulin and glucose levels during and following exercise can be more safely managed.

- The possibility of combining with a CGM and the Threshold (Low Glucose) Suspend System or a Predicted Low Glucose Suspend System offers safety in the prevention of hypoglycemia (see Chapter 30). This involves turning a pump off for up to two hours when the CGM detects or predicts a low glucose level. Time spent with low blood sugars, particularly at night, is reduced as a result. The era of the artificial pancreas has now begun (see Chapter 30) and requires use of an insulin pump and a CGM.

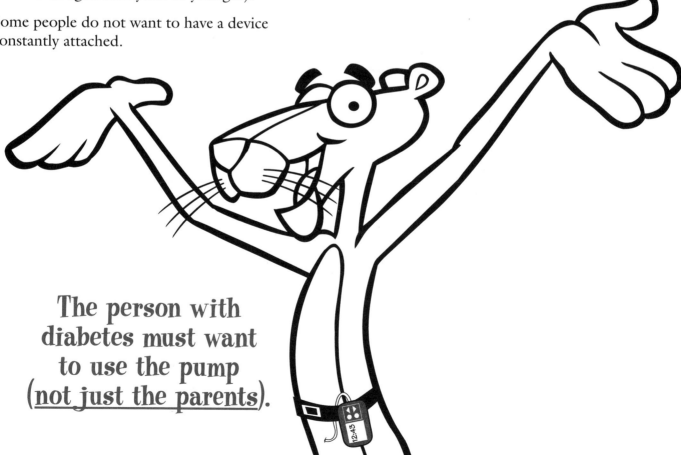

The person with diabetes must want to use the pump (not just the parents).

Using an insulin pump
sometimes increases
one's energy.

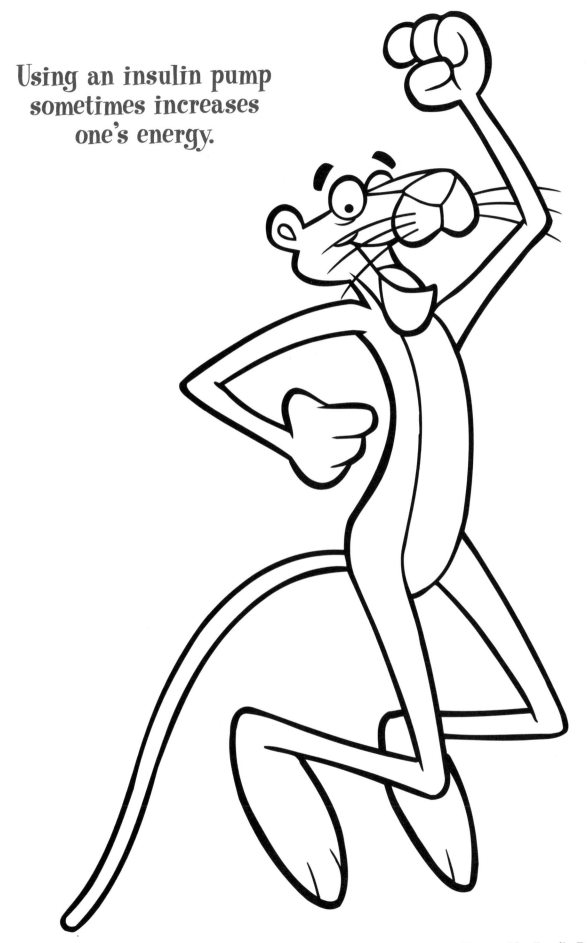

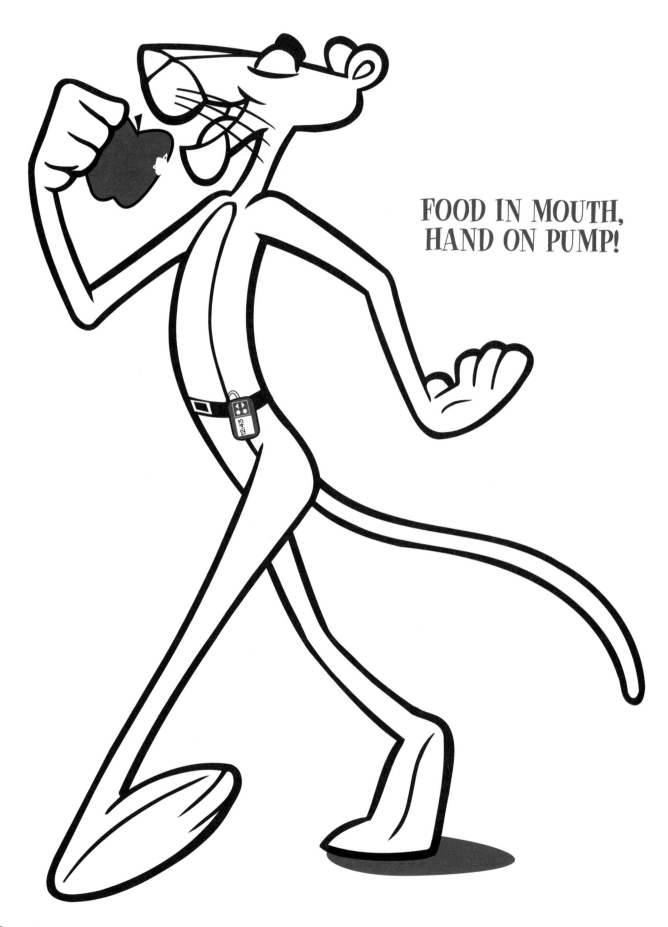

FOOD IN MOUTH,
HAND ON PUMP!

Chapter 29
Continuous Glucose Monitors (CGM)

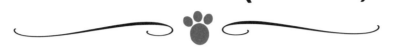

Continuous glucose monitors (CGM) give readings of subcutaneous (the tissue under the skin) glucose levels every five minutes. This compares with finger-stick blood sugar (glucose) readings which are often done only four to six times each day. The subcutaneous CGM glucose values are approximately 10 minutes behind the blood sugar values. This is because the sugar must pass through the blood vessel wall into the subcutaneous space, and then the CGM system must determine the value. This delay is not clinically important unless the blood glucose is changing rapidly.

In 2016, the FDA approved the MiniMed/Medtronic 670G Hybrid Artificial Pancreas system. The CGM glucose values are sent to the insulin pump which contains formulas to increase, decrease, stop or start insulin administration as needed to control sugar levels (see Chapter 30). The CGM is an important part of the artificial pancreas.

The FDA has approved insulin dosing using the Dexcom G5 or G6 and the FreeStyle Libre Flash CGMs. The Dexcom G6 does not require calibration (no finger-sticks), can be worn for 10 days, has a simple one-touch sensor insertion and is not affected by acetaminophen (e.g., Tylenol). These devices make care for children, especially in the school setting, much easier. We recommend finger stick blood sugars for verification of low CGM sugar values and for following the rise in blood sugar levels after treatment. We also recommend doing a finger-stick blood sugar in the school setting if the CGM value is below 80 (4.5) or above 250 (13.9) mg/dL (mmol/L). The Dexcom G6, when available, will not have interference from acetaminophen and may not require twice-daily finger stick blood sugars for calibration.

In 2017, the Abbot FreeStyle Libre "Flash" was approved by the FDA. The sensor is small (~the size of two quarters) and transmits glucose values to a monitor when it is waved over the sensor. Finger-stick blood glucose calibrations are not required. The sensor can be worn for 10 days (14 in Europe) and there is no interference from acetaminophen. The monitor shows a graph of scanned glucose values and has rate of change arrows. It does not have warning alarms for low or high glucose values.

The purpose of this chapter is to present a brief overview of CGM. An entire book is available for people wanting detailed information (*"Understanding Insulin Pumps, Continuous Glucose Monitors and the Artificial Pancreas" – see ordering materials in the back of this book*). Some essential points of CGM use are summarized below.

- The person, and not just the parents, must want to use the CGM (except for the very young).

- Currently, finger-stick blood sugar levels may or may not be required (depending on the device). Finger-stick blood sugars are still recommended anytime a low or high blood sugar is suspected, or if the CGM value is in question.

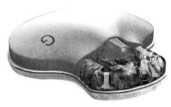

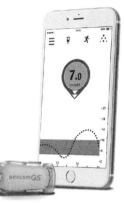

- The CGM values will not always match the blood sugar values.

- The more the CGM is worn, the more it can help.

- For some devices, the CGM glucose values can be sent "via the cloud" to a phone, watch or other device of parents or other providers. This can be very comforting to parents of young children.

THE COMPONENTS OF A CGM

All CGMs have three basic parts:

1. Sensor: As with the insulin pump, a tiny probe is inserted (with the push of a button) under the skin. The sensor reads subcutaneous (not blood) glucose levels for the next six or seven days (it is often possible to make them last even longer).

2. Transmitter: The transmitter attaches to or is built into the sensor and sends the glucose reading to the receiver (which can be a device, smart phone or pump). For some CGMs, the transmitter can also transmit the reading via "the cloud" to be viewed on a phone, watch or other commercial device.

3. Receiver or Monitor: The receiver receives the glucose readings from the transmitter. It is a mini-computer that can record and save weeks of glucose information. Several systems now have the receiver within the insulin pump, and the readings are viewable on the pump's screen.

INITIATING CGM THERAPY

As with initiation of an insulin pump, various clinics will have different protocols for beginning CGM therapy. The criteria for deciding who is ready to begin CGM therapy are similar to those discussed for starting an insulin pump (Chapter 28). Many clinics also have CGM systems for short-term and/or diagnostic use.

SOME ADVANTAGES OF CGM

Glucose levels: Knowing glucose levels every few minutes throughout the day, particularly after meals and during the night, can be a great help. Knowing the average glucose level is also helpful in long-term glucose control.

Trend graphs: The trend graphs show the direction a glucose level is going (in contrast to a single point in time for a blood sugar level).

Rate of Change Arrows: These arrows can help to alert that a rapid change in glucose levels is occurring. Some people use these arrows to help guide insulin bolus dosing (See *"Understanding Diabetes"* and *"Understanding Insulin Pumps, CGMs and the Artificial Pancreas"* for more information on this topic).

Warning alarms: The alarms for high and low glucose levels (or pending levels) can help to prevent episodes of DKA or hypoglycemia.

Preventing severe hypoglycemia: The first part of the artificial pancreas (Chapter 30) was approved for the U.S. by the FDA in September, 2013. It is called the "Artificial Pancreas Device System," or the 530-G (or 630-G) Threshold (Low Glucose) Suspend System. A Predicted Low Glucose Suspend System is also available which helps to prevent hypoglycemia before it occurs. It is present in the Hybrid Artificial Pancreas (see below) as well as other devices in development. These systems involve the pump turning off insulin infusion for up to two hours when the CGM detects a low or predicts a low glucose level will occur. The MiniMed/Medtronic 670G Hybrid Artificial Pancreas system, using the MiniMed CGM, was approved by the FDA in 2016 (see above and Chapter 30). It increases time with glucose levels in-range and reduces the time spent with low glucose levels.

Reduced finger pokes: Fewer blood sugars are generally needed.

Lower HbA1c: If worn consistently (e.g., six days per week), HbA1c levels usually decrease.

SOME ISSUES WITH CGM

Adhesive issues: Adhesion issues for the sensor/transmitter are one of the two most frequent difficulties with CGM. For some people this is not a problem. For others, it is a major difficulty. The issues are discussed in detail in the Pump, CGM and Artificial Pancreas book referred to above.

Calibration: A second issue with CGM involves calibrating the system so that the CGM values are as accurate as possible and are matching the blood sugar values. Calibration involves doing a finger-stick blood sugar and entering it into the receiver, preferably at a time when the blood sugar is not rapidly changing. Not all CGM systems require calibration.

Alarms: Some people are annoyed by the alarms for high and low glucose levels or for the need to do a calibration. Alarms can be set on higher or lower glucose levels to help in making them less frequent, or on "vibrate," or can be turned off. If bothersome, discuss with the diabetes care-providers.

Comfort: Although some people have in the past found the sensors to be uncomfortable due to their bulk, they have gradually gotten smaller.

Cost: Insurance coverage should be checked prior to ordering the CGM system. Coverage is gradually improving.

Accuracy: As with development of blood sugar meters, each new sensor version is more accurate. There will always be occasional sensors that do not function well.

SENSOR PLACEMENT AND ADHESION

Placement: Each CGM company has suggestions for where to place their sensors. In general, they can be worn on the back of the arm, the abdomen, hips, or buttocks. The selected area must have enough skin/fat to be able to pinch up a little bit with two fingers.

Adhesive use: There are many different adhesive wipes, tapes, and bandages that can help sensors to stick to skin. It is quite common for a person to use an adhesive wipe to treat the skin under the sensor, to then place the sensor on the skin, and finally to reinforce it with additional tape. Every person is different, and what works for one person may not work for others. Detailed suggestions are given in the Pump, CGM and Artificial Pancreas book.

CGM DATA

There are two main types of data that can be obtained from CGM usage: **Real-Time** and **Retrospective**. **Real-time** data refers to data available while wearing the CGM, such as a "trend-graph" showing a series of glucose values. Arrows showing the rate of change can also be very helpful. **Retrospective** data refers to data from the past, most often downloaded using a computer. Both types of data are important and are explained in detail in the Pump, CGM and Artificial Pancreas book.

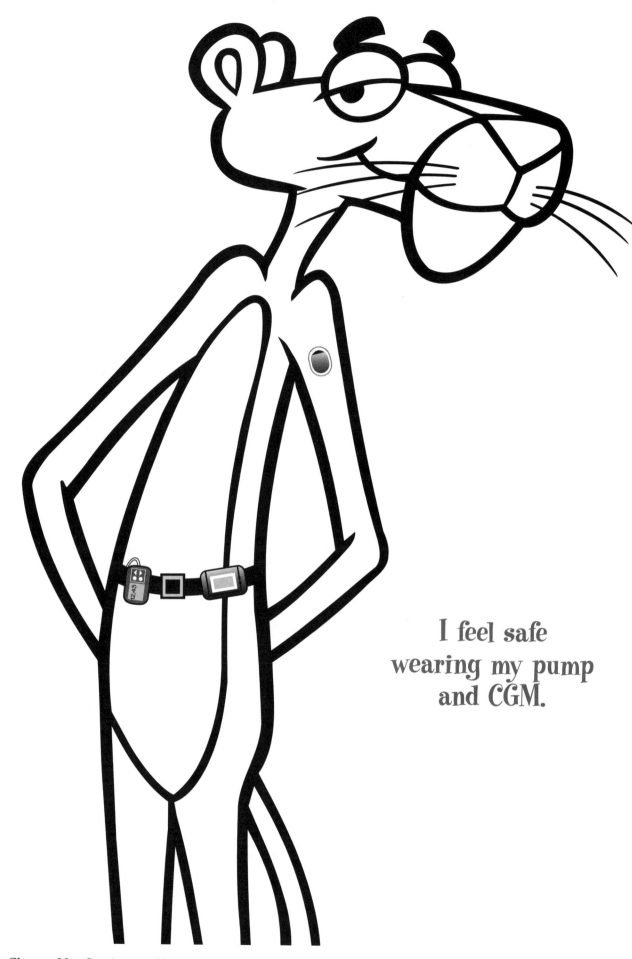

I feel safe
wearing my pump
and CGM.

Chapter 30
The Artificial Pancreas

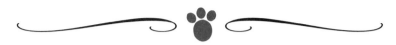

The artificial pancreas ("Closed loop pancreas" or "Automated insulin delivery") refers to a combination of a continuous glucose monitor (CGM) and an insulin pump working together to increase, decrease, stop or start insulin administration as needed to control blood glucose levels. The CGM sends the glucose data to the pump where mathematical formulas (algorithms) tell the pump how to regulate the insulin. The artificial pancreas was approved in September, 2016, and became commercially available in 2017. Various forms of the artificial pancreas will gradually become the "treatment of choice" for type 1 diabetes.

Severe hypoglycemia is dangerous, and the ability to stop an insulin infusion from an insulin pump with a low CGM glucose level, or even better, with an impending low CGM glucose level, is very important. Approximately half of severe hypoglycemic events in adults and 75 percent in children occur during sleep. Thus, decreasing basal insulin or turning a pump off with actual or predicted hypoglycemia during the night is extremely valuable. Warning alarms are also valuable, but frequently do not awaken people during the night.

High blood sugar levels are also not good for the brain. The complete artificial pancreas will provide extra insulin with high glucose levels to reduce the time spent with high blood sugar. The time spent "in-range" (often considered 70-180 mg/dL [3.9-10 mmol/L]) is consistently increased, especially at night. The wide swings in glucose levels are also reduced.

I) PARTIAL ARTIFICIAL PANCREAS SYSTEMS
THRESHOLD SUSPEND, SUSPEND ON LOW, OR LOW GLUCOSE SUSPEND (all the same)

The Threshold Suspend, (referred to outside the U.S. as Low Glucose Suspend [LGS]), a feature of the Medtronic Sensor Augmented Pump System, is available within and outside the U.S. This requires use of the Medtronic 530G or 630G insulin pump and the Enlite sensor with the Medtronic CGM. Outside the U.S., the system uses the Paradigm VEO insulin pump and the Low Glucose Suspend feature.

The Threshold Suspend system represented a major advancement in the development of the artificial pancreas. The insulin pump is turned off for up to two hours if the CGM glucose value is below a set level (often 60 mg/dL or 3.3 mmol/L). The person can respond to the alarm, consume carbs, and turn the pump back on at any time during the two hours. This is what occurs in the majority of cases, particularly during the day. Most of the full two-hour suspensions (with alarms not responded to by the wearer) occur during sleep. This feature has been shown in multiple research reports to reduce time spent in hypoglycemia. There is also some evidence that wearing the Threshold Suspend System will reduce the number of lows. **Most important, it is an effective therapy to help prevent severe hypoglycemic episodes.**

PREDICTED LOW GLUCOSE SUSPEND (PLGS)

It is obviously better to prevent hypoglycemia than to treat it (e.g., stopping pump insulin delivery before hypoglycemia occurs). In addition to the person feeling better, the body does not reduce stores of adrenaline (epinephrine). By predicting that the glucose level is going to become low, the pump can decrease or stop insulin to prevent the low, or at least to reduce the duration of the low sugar level. Current overnight data suggests a glucose level must be below 60 mg/dL (3.3 mmol/L) for over two hours before a hypoglycemic seizure would occur. Use of the PLGS (and of the LGS) can greatly reduce the risk that this would occur. This feature is a part of the MiniMed/Medtronic 670G artificial pancreas. Some other insulin pump manufacturers will likely soon have this feature prior to moving to a complete artificial pancreas system.

II) THE HYBRID AND/OR COMPLETE ARTIFICIAL PANCREAS SYSTEM

The artificial pancreas is described in the Introduction of this chapter. The initial version of the artificial pancreas (Medtronic 670G Hybrid Closed Loop System) is called a "hybrid" artificial pancreas because it is still recommended that pre-meal insulin boluses be administered by the user 20 to 30 minutes prior to meals. This is because blood sugar levels peak 60 minutes after meals, but insulin activity does not peak until 90 minutes after injection (see Figure in Chapter 8). High blood sugar levels develop after meals if a person/family does not do the pre-meal bolus, and the insulin is only given by the insulin pump after the CGM glucose levels rise. Also, when this happens, low blood sugar levels may be more apt to occur two to four hours after the meal. As better ultra-rapid-acting insulins are developed, pre-meal insulin administration will not be necessary and the word "hybrid" will no longer be necessary.

Although the Medtronic 670G hybrid artificial pancreas was the first system made available in the U.S., other companies will likely follow. The Tandem pump will use the Dexcom CGM with a low glucose suspend and PLGS system to help prevent hypoglycemia (expected to be available in late 2018 or early 2019). The "Bigfoot Biomedical" company will use the Asante pump and is partnering with Abbott to have a sensor in the system that does not require calibration. The "Beta Bionic" company (Boston University) has the iLet device with a dual chamber for insulin and glucagon. The University of Cambridge has used the Abbott Navigator CGM and the Abbott Florence pump. The Insulet Omnipod will use the Dexcom in their system. The Inreada system from the Netherlands may be an early system to be available in Europe. Thus, with time, other artificial pancreas systems will likely become available.

With the artificial pancreas, sugar control will be greatly improved, with reduced danger of severe hypoglycemia, a reduction of high glucose levels and more glucose values in the desired range. Although people will need to remain diligent in self-care, overall management will be safer and easier.

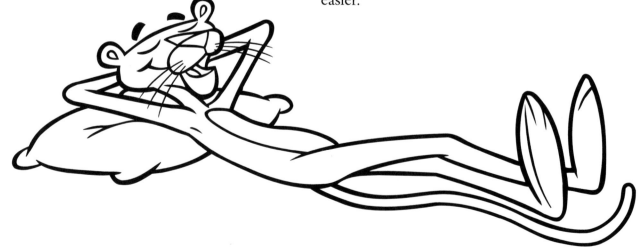

Chapter 31
Pregnancy and Diabetes

Pregnancy is possible for women with diabetes who do not have severe problems with complications. Pregnancy is discussed in more detail in the book *"Management of Diabetes in Adults"* (see ordering materials in the back of this book).

WHAT IS IMPORTANT WHEN THINKING ABOUT GETTING PREGNANT?

- Pregnancy should be planned, in order to minimize risk to mother and baby.

- The best sugar control possible should be achieved before and during pregnancy. The HbA1c should be below 6.5% (48 mmol/mol). (The ADA recommends below 6.0% [42 mmol/mol].)

- The risk of a miscarriage, as well as birth defects in the baby, are less if blood/CGM sugar values are normal or near normal when the pregnancy begins. This is why it is recommend to plan a pregnancy only after tight sugar control has been achieved.

- Some medications commonly used in people with diabetes have been implicated in causing birth defects. Examples of these are drugs for blood pressure and kidney protection (example: ACE inhibitors) and cholesterol lowering drugs (statins). You should discuss use of any of these medications with your physician before becoming pregnant.

- Folic acid should be taken for three months before the pregnancy to also help prevent birth defects.

HOW CAN THE BEST SUGAR CONTROL BE ACHIEVED?

Intensive insulin therapy is usual during pregnancy. This includes:

- An insulin pump or frequent insulin shots

- Frequent blood sugar checks (eight to ten a day) or use of a CGM

- Paying close attention to nutrition

- Frequent contact with the healthcare team

The target values for blood/CGM sugar values are lower than usual and are given in the Table in Chapter 15 of the above referenced book *"Management of Diabetes in Adults."*

Clinic visits are also more frequent, usually every two to four weeks.

WHAT ABOUT COMPLICATIONS AND PREGNANCY?

Kidney damage is usually not a problem during pregnancy unless already present before the pregnancy. Medicines used to prevent kidney damage called "ACE inhibitors" should not be taken during pregnancy. This medicine could cause birth defects in the baby.

The eyes should be checked more often during pregnancy (at least every three months). If moderate damage is already present, this may get worse during pregnancy.

GESTATIONAL DIABETES

Gestational diabetes is diabetes that develops as a result of the stress of the pregnancy. Regular exercise and diet are important.

- After diagnosis, care during pregnancy is similar to that of a person who had diabetes prior to pregnancy.

- Gestational diabetes usually goes away after pregnancy. Women who have gestational diabetes have an increased risk of developing type 2 diabetes later in life.

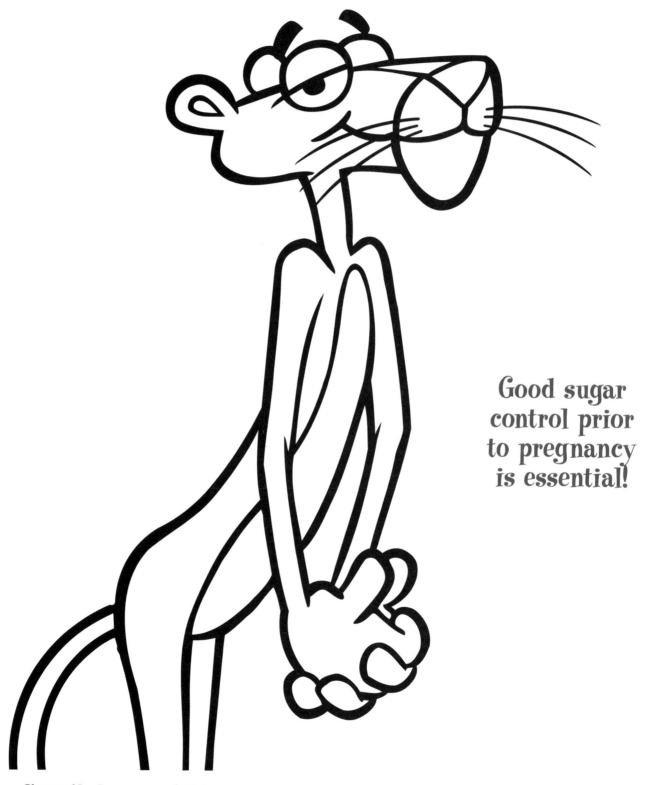

Good sugar control prior to pregnancy is essential!

Chapter 32
Research and Diabetes

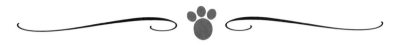

THE FIVE MOST FREQUENTLY ASKED QUESTIONS RELATE TO:

A Cure

Pancreas or islet transplantation is already possible. The problem is that the strong medicines necessary to prevent rejection can be more harmful than having diabetes. Many new medicines are being tried, but it is still early. Stem cell research is now progressing and may, in the future, provide a source of islets capable of physiologic insulin production.

The Artificial Pancreas

In 2016, the FDA approved the MiniMed/Medtronic 670G Hybrid Artificial Pancreas system. The CGM glucose values are sent to the insulin pump, which contains formulas to increase, decrease, stop or start insulin administration as needed to control sugar levels (see Chapter 30). The CGM and the insulin pump are important parts of the artificial pancreas. With time, other artificial pancreas systems will become available. A book, *"Understanding Insulin Pumps, Continuous Glucose Monitors and the Artificial Pancreas"* is available for those wanting more information (see ordering materials in the back of this book).

Prevention of Type 1 Diabetes (see www.diabetestrialnet.org)

- Several trials are currently under way to attempt to find ways to prevent type 1 diabetes.

- Four biochemical islet cell antibodies (Chapter 3) are being used to determine whether the autoimmune process has begun.

- People with a relative with type 1 diabetes may be eligible for a free TrialNet islet antibody screening (more information at www.trialnet.org, or in the U.S., call 1-800-425-8361).

- Children from the general population (no relatives with type 1 diabetes) in Colorado, U.S.A., (Autoimmunity Screening for Kids: askhealth.org) and Germany (Fr1da study) are also being screened for islet autoantibodies. These studies may eventually lead to more widespread screening for type 1 diabetes risk, but this is not yet standard care.

- If there are islet antibodies (signs of autoimmunity), people may be eligible for research trials to try to reverse the process and prevent diabetes.

- Prevention trials are now focused on:

  ~ preventing the autoimmune process from starting

  ~ reversing the autoimmune process to prevent diabetes

  ~ stopping further damage to the islets after diabetes has been diagnosed (to extend the "honeymoon")

Prevention of Type 2 Diabetes

- This has already been shown to be possible.

- It usually involves eating less, exercising more, and losing weight.

- It is discussed in Chapter 4 of *"Understanding Diabetes."*

Prevention of Complications

- Diabetes complications are decreasing through attention being paid to the following:

  ~ better sugar control

  ~ exercise, a healthy diet and optimal body weight

  ~ blood pressure control

  ~ not smoking

  ~ normal levels of blood lipids (e.g., total cholesterol and LDL cholesterol)

  ~ regular eye exams and urine microalbumin levels (to check the kidneys). These should be initiated for people who have had type 1 diabetes for five or more years, starting at age 10 years or at puberty, whichever is first (see Chapter 23). People with type 2 diabetes should have initial evaluations at the time of diagnosis. The evaluations should then be repeated annually or at intervals as recommended by their diabetes care-providers.

- Research is also looking at ways to slow or stop complications in people who have early signs of kidney or eye damage.

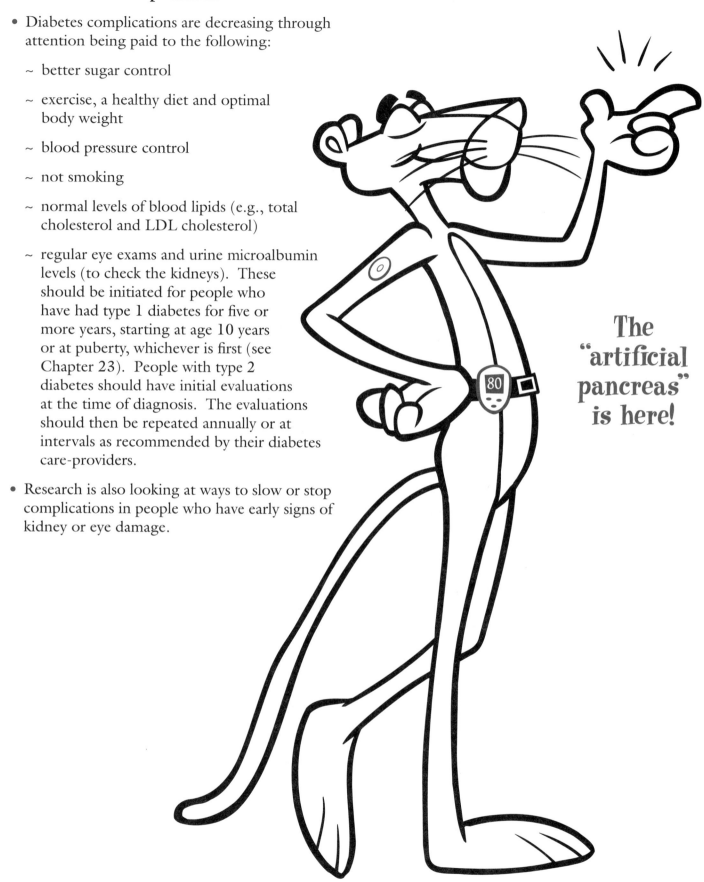

The "artificial pancreas" is here!

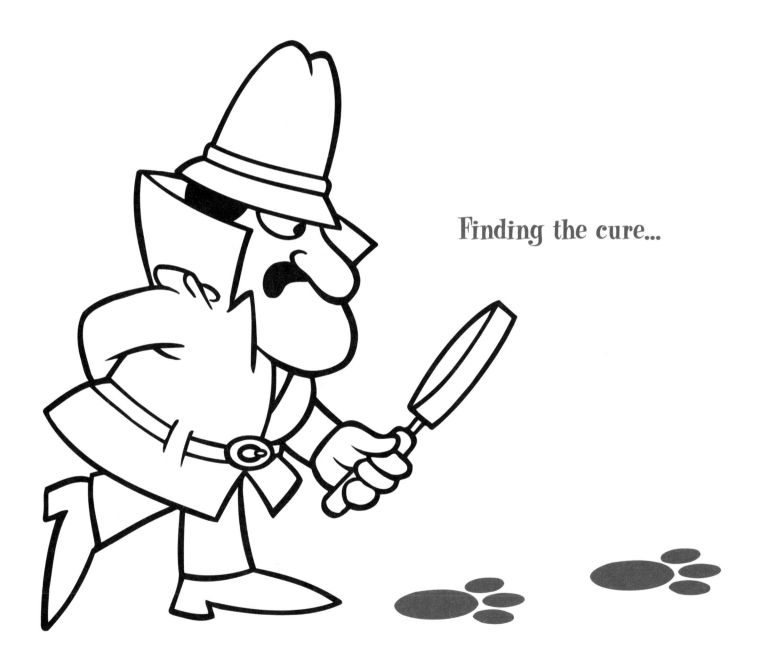

Finding the cure...

Someday there will be
A CURE FOR DIABETES!

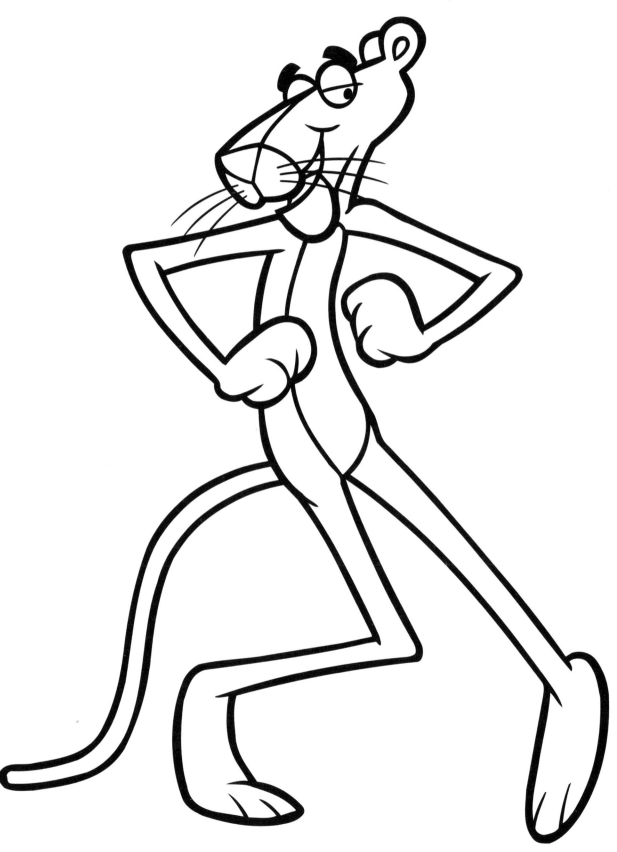

Publications

Additional copies of "A First Book for Understanding Diabetes" as well as other diabetes publications may be ordered by using this form, by calling the Children's Diabetes Foundation at 303-863-1200, or by visiting our website at www.ChildrensDiabetesFoundation.org

Children's Diabetes Foundation
4380 South Syracuse Street, Suite 430 • Denver, CO 80237

Name: _____

Address: _____

City, State, ZIP: _____

Phone:_____ Email: _____

Quantity	Item	Price	Total
	A First Book for Understanding Diabetes, 14th Edition Presents the essentials from *Understanding Diabetes*	$15.00*	
	Un Primer Libro Para Entender La Diabetes 14th Edition	$15.00*	
	Understanding Diabetes – "The Pink Panther Book" 13th Edition	$25.00*	
	Insulin Pumps, Continuous Glucose Monitors and the Artificial Pancreas, 3rd Edition	$18.00*	
	Management of Diabetes in Adults, 1st Edition	$15.00*	
	DIABETES: A History of a Center and a Patient	$15.00*	
	A Cure — A novel about diabetes and the search for a cure	$20.00*	
	Residents of the State of Colorado add 7.75% sales tax		
	SHIPPING AND HANDLING: $5.00 per book for orders of 1-9 books $2.00 per book for orders of 10 books and over	Shipping and Handling	
		TOTAL	

* Prices subject to change.

☐ Please include me on the Children's Diabetes Foundation mailing list.

☐ Check enclosed payable to: Children's Diabetes Foundation

☐ Visa ☐ MasterCard ☐ Discovery ☐ AmEx

Card # _____Exp. Date _____

All orders must be paid in full before we can mail. Books are mailed USPS or Ground UPS.
Allow one to three weeks for delivery.

Canadian and Foreign Purchasers: Please include sufficient funds
to equal U.S. currency exchange rates.

For quantity order pricing and additional information call 303-863-1200 or visit our website at
www.ChildrensDiabetesFoundation.org

Websites

Barbara Davis Center for Diabetes
University of Colorado Denver
Mail Stop A140, Building M20
1775 Aurora Court
Aurora, CO 80045
303-724-2323 • Fax 303-724-6779
www.BarbaraDavisCenter.org

Children's Diabetes Foundation
www.ChildrensDiabetesFoundation.org

Children With Diabetes
www.ChildrenWithDiabetes.com

Juvenile Diabetes Research Foundation
www.jdrf.org

American Diabetes Association
www.diabetes.org